God Knows
You're
Stressed

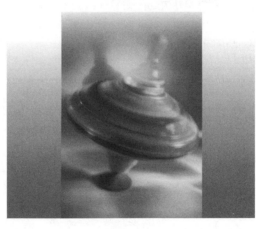

God Knows
You're
Stressed

Simple ways to restore your balance

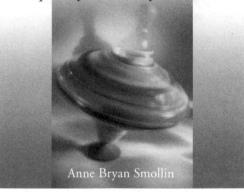

Anne Bryan Smollin

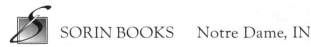 SORIN BOOKS   Notre Dame, IN

www.sorinbooks.com

ISBN-10 1-893732-35-5   ISBN-13 978-1-893732-35-3

Cover and text design by Katherine Robinson Coleman

Printed and bound in the United States of America.

Library of Congress Cataloging-in-Publication Data
Smollin, Anne Bryan.
     God knows you're stressed : simple ways to restore your balance / Anne Bryan Smollin.
          p. cm.
     ISBN 1-893732-35-5
     1. Stress (Psychology)--Religious aspects--Christianity. 2. Stress management. I. Title.
     RA785 .S67 2001
     155.9'042--dc21

                                                            2001002435
                                                            CIP

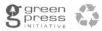

CONTENTS

Introduction

Yes, as you may have guessed, there is plenty of bad news associated with stress.

Stress, by definition, is the inability to cope with a real or imagined threat to our well-being, which results in a series of responses and adaptations by our bodies. Stress makes us exhausted, fatigued, angry, and anxious.

Stress does not always directly cause illness, but it has been proven to be a contributing factor. Physical conditions like indigestion, diarrhea, ulcers, poor appetite, bronchitis, pneumonia, sweating, chest pains, muscle aches, frequent colds, and trembling have been attributed at least in part to stress. Stress has also been linked to migraines, asthma, psoriasis, hives, allergies, irritable bowel syndrome, eczema, heart disease, and high blood pressure.

Stress causes cholesterol to rise as much or more than does diet. The dread of going to work and the excitement about getting away from work stress the body. So, irregular heartbeats (arrhythmia) peak on Mondays and Fridays. Americans make 187 million visits to doctors each year for stress-related complaints. One study shows that by the age of six years old, many of us have already laid the groundwork for severe high blood pressure.

Mental symptoms like lack of concentration, poor memory, confusion, forgetfulness, and lack of humor are red flags, indicating a high level of stress. Emotionally, a stressed-out person may experience anger, depression, hopelessness, irritability, fearfulness, powerlessness, guilt, or shame. And behaviorally, highly stressed people tend to throw things, swear, yell, hit, bite their nails, tap their feet, cry, and fidget more often.

Unmanaged stress is a higher risk factor for cancer and heart disease than either cigarette smoking or high cholesterol foods. Studies show us that one million people in this country are absent from work each day because of stress-related disorders.

Little children may experience stress when they have no one to play with or when their favorite toy is broken. A teenager may experience stress when she or he is thrown out of a group or feels different or out of place. A college student may feel stressed when the pressure of studies becomes unbearable.

There are typically three levels of stress. The first level stressors are mild or brief: missing our bus, misplacing concert tickets, or breaking a glass. At the time this incident occurs we feel frustration and anxiety. However, the stress is situational.

Moderate-level stress is harder to deal with. Preparing for a wedding, unmet deadlines at work that require overtime, significant people being away for a short period of time, and adjusting to a child going away to college are some common causes of moderate stress. These take more of our energy, and consequently stress stays in our body longer.

Finally, there is the chronic or severe stress level that is related to going through a divorce, the loss of a significant person, the death of a spouse, child, or a loved one. This level of stress may require us to seek outside help and support.

Had enough of the bad news about stress?

Now the Good News

Stress does not have to bring us down! The things that happen to us do not cause stress. Rather it is our reaction to what happens that causes the stress. We have the power to choose how we react to stress. Our attitudes determine our choices, and our choices can determine our attitudes. Hence, we are in control of the stress in our own lives.

God Knows You're Stressed: Simple Ways to Restore Your Balance offers proven advice, inspiring stories, and useful activities to help recover the balance that we all desire. Stress can be transformed. We can learn to cope with stress and even grow healthier in the process. Good news indeed.

Using the Book

God Knows You're Stressed: Simple Ways to Restore Your Balance is a book to make your way through slowly, thoughtfully, and actively. Keep it by your bed; read a section at night before you drift off to sleep. Spend several days pondering a story or repeating one of the activities. Post one of the short sayings on your bathroom mirror, so that every time you look there you can remind yourself about one of the basic ways of managing stress.

In other words, take your time. It has taken years for most of us to reach the level of stress we are at. We have developed habits that contribute to our stress. Habits take time to transform.

Use this book to help you with this transformation. Page by page, may you learn to like yourself better, treat yourself with more kindness, laugh more, play more, breathe more deeply, rest more soundly, and hold hurts more loosely. May your reading and reflection bring health, balance, and a richer life.

WAY 1 :

Decide to Be Imperfect

HE WHO HAS NEVER FAILED
SOMEWHERE, THAT MAN CANNOT
BE GREAT.

Herman Melville

W̲ho ever said we have to be perfect? Aiming for perfection—whatever that means—puts us in a no-win, highly stressful situation. After all, humans cannot possibly be perfect. Perfection is not part of our human nature. Much evidence abounds about our imperfection. For example, one study showed that an average American spends one year of his or her lifetime searching for misplaced objects. We forget items, make mistakes, say the wrong thing, and generally mess up. We're not even close to being perfect. So, to escape this stress-producing vice, start by deciding to be *imperfect*!

Remember when you learned to ride a bicycle or to drive a car? You didn't master these skills immediately. You felt clumsy and awkward. You didn't feel dumb or stupid. You knew you had to learn to balance yourself on the bike and pedal and steer. You knew you had to learn to check the rear-view and side mirrors of the car.

You had to learn to stay on your own side of the road and judge distances with other cars. You knew that you had to learn.

Learning to drive or to maneuver a bike was a process. Once you mastered these skills, you likely forgot the mistakes and the clumsy, awkward feelings. Once you mastered the skills, you no longer thought about adjusting seats and mirrors. The skills were now second nature to you.

There is no such thing as instant success. Success is based on many attempts and many re-doings. A Spanish proverb teaches: "However early you get up, you cannot hasten the dawn." Thomas Edison took over a thousand tries to discover which filament to use for the incandescent light bulb.

We block ourselves from taking on new endeavors because we are afraid of failure, so we settle into mediocrity. Sadness comes from giving up or from letting the mistakes and failures block our successes. Hockey great Wayne Gretzky remarked that "we miss one hundred percent of the shots we never take." And Isaac Newton declared, "No great discovery was ever made without a bold guess."

When we are still learning or when new challenges present themselves, we can rely on our creativity to get matters accomplished—to boldly guess. I recall a situation in which I was totally helpless and had no idea what I was supposed to do. I entered the Sisters of Saint Joseph, a community of Catholic sisters, when I was seventeen years old. We lived in a building that one would call a college dorm. There were a total of 135 living in the house. We did the cooking, cleaning, carpentry, plumbing, and whatever else was needed to care for the building.

One day, while I was taking my turn at cooking, the person in charge had to leave the kitchen. I was going solo, and it was my responsibility to see that the lunch would be served on time. The supervisor told me to make tapioca pudding. I had placed all the contents in a large pot. She instructed me to put it in a double boiler. Then she left for her meeting. I had no idea what a double boiler was. There was no one I could ask. So I placed the huge pot between two burners and began stirring.

Eventually the one in charge returned and rescued the tapioca pudding. At the rate it was cooking on the two burners, the pudding would not have been ready for Christmas! I learned what a double boiler was, the group had dessert, and I moved forward from the experience.

If we can be imperfect, we can be ourselves. We can accept good qualities and rough edges, our strengths and weaknesses, and not be paralyzed by our ineptitude. When we celebrate our giftedness as well as our limitations, we embrace our life as whole. Not perfect, but whole. Loving ourselves means loving all of who we are.

And we must also *like* ourselves. Liking is different from loving. Liking implies knowing and caring for ourselves. It implies being gentle with ourselves. Until this happens we operate out of a deficit of healthy, creative living. We will lose spontaneity and limit our own abilities. We will discount any newness and never learn to play or relax or enjoy ourselves. Deciding to accept imperfection—our humanity—takes a lot of weight off of our shoulders and stress out of our life.

IF YOU THINK YOU CAN, OR YOU
THINK YOU CANNOT, YOU'RE
ALWAYS RIGHT.

Henry Ford

Decide to Be Imperfect

• Enjoy your imperfection by:

- For a week, keep track of mistakes that you make. Instead of beating yourself up for them, acknowledge each one and consciously forgive yourself by saying something like, "I rejoice in my humanity and like myself, mistakes and all!"

- Note instances each day when you did not know how to do something or when you asked a question. Celebrate your ignorance as opportunities to learn. Start embracing imperfection as positive chances to grow.

- Memorize this principle: "Things worth doing are worth doing poorly." Instead of thinking that we have to do everything or the whole job, we need to teach ourselves that it is possible and healthy to just use whatever time we have available to us. We look out at our gardens and think that we have to go and pull out all the weeds. Why don't we just pull out the big ones? When we are having company, we think we have to polish all the silverware. Why don't we just polish what we are going to use that evening?

- Think about something you did recently that you considered a mistake. How did you feel? What did you do about your feeling? What did you learn from the whole incident? It is important for us to see that positive things often are the result of what we call our "mistakes." So often something better happens than we could have first imagined.

- Try something that you have never done before or stopped doing because someone told you that it was silly: Stand in the living room and dance ai ng with the music on the radio. Experiment with a recipe; make changes that feel right to you. Find a computer application on your home computer that you have never used; try it and see what happens. Take up a new sport that you have always wanted to try; become a clumsy beginner and enjoy your mistakes. If you are afraid, know that we are all afraid of doing things we've never done before. That's natural! If you're frightened, do it frightened. Remember that you fell down the first time you tried to walk, but that didn't let you stop from trying again. In failing, we learn what doesn't work.

> THERE ARE TWO MISTAKES ONE CAN
> MAKE ALONG THE ROAD TO TRUTH:
> NOT GOING ALL THE WAY, AND NOT
> STARTING.
>
> *Siddhartha Gautama*

Running

I know it sounds crazy, but depression got my life into some kind of balance. Treatment actually freed me from the terrible stress of having to be a success, having to be perfect all the time, in everything. That I spent most of my life struggling under the weight of perfectionism saddens and amazes me. My head knew I didn't have to be a champion in everything, but the rest of me just didn't go along. When I got seriously depressed, I suddenly realized how I had to get rid of that unconscious drive to be perfect or I would probably never crawl out of the darkness and distress.

While talking my way through the depression, two stories stuck out in my mind about how driven I was. This is where the sadness comes in. I denied myself some opportunities for growth because I always had to be the best. I especially felt this way in high school.

I was a miler on the track team. I set a conference record for freshmen, improved as a sophomore, and had an unbeaten streak going as a junior when I met a kid that I'll name Taylor. He came from a family of top-notch runners. For the first three laps I kept behind him. As soon as the bell rang for the final lap, he took off. I was running the best race of my life, and he just buried me. At that moment I decided that I could never beat him. The feeling was terrible. And it only got worse.

During my senior year, I was running well again. But I knew that Taylor was out there, burning up everyone he faced. Districts approached. To go to the state finals I had to run in the districts. Taylor wouldn't be there, but I knew he would bury me again at state. I couldn't face that. So, I took the only way out that I could think of.

I had not been feeling too great, but I had run well feeling a lot worse. Anyway, I went to a doctor for a checkup. Actually, I knew this doctor didn't approve of the hard training schedule our coach put us through. I also knew that he would give me an excuse to get out of running at practice. And also out of the district meet. Looking back now, I know that unconsciously I just couldn't face Taylor again and get buried. Living with the knowledge that I didn't even try was still better than facing defeat at Taylor's hands. What a lost opportunity.

Over my lifetime I have pulled away from many good experiences because I decided that I couldn't be perfect or successful. One other example has proven a particular handicap. Here I am in the age of computers, but I can't type. I had a chance to take typing, also as a high school senior, but decided not to. My grade point average was a perfect 4.0—all A's for four years. My fine motor skills being what they were, I was afraid that I would get less than an A and not be valedictorian if I took typing. Sure enough, I became the valedictorian who couldn't type. I had a perfect GPA, but not a basic, useful skill. Another lost opportunity.

Life has been good, don't get me wrong. Even so, it has actually gotten a lot better since I decided after the depression that I didn't have to be the best. Now I run for fun, but I still have to get things typed for me.

Vincent Hatt

IT TAKES COURAGE TO GROW UP
AND TURN OUT TO BE
WHO YOU REALLY ARE.

e. e. cummings

Tom's Story

Tom, a forty-one-year-old man, was dying of AIDS. His family was in total denial. His parents literally had him locked in an upstairs bedroom. They did care for his basic necessities like food and water, thank heavens.

The first time I visited Tom at his parents' home, I was brought up to his bedroom. This huge, handsome man was now terribly thin and looked lost in the king-sized bed. I bent over to kiss him and then sat beside his bed. I took his hand and said, "Now tell me what you want me to know."

"No one touches me anymore."

I continued holding his hand and let him unravel his story.

After several visits at his home, Tom became so ill that it was necessary to hospitalize him. Each day after work, I would drive over to visit with him in the hospital. I would try to engage his mother and father in conversation. Nothing seemed to work. Knowing it was therapeutic for all of them to be able to talk about Tom's condition, I tried many different techniques. I was successful with his brother and sister-in-law, but the parents had built high walls around the subject. Meanwhile, Tom's condition worsened daily.

After about five weeks, the family seemed to look forward to my arrival at the hospital each day. There were times I spent alone with Tom. He wanted and needed to tell me other pieces of his story. He was a wonderful man who had made one choice that left its mark on him. Apparently he felt safe with me. I did not judge him. We found things to laugh at and, at times, the laughter coming from his room brought smiles to those passing in the corridor.

Tom feared that he had been a failure. Though everyone who knew him described Tom as generous, kind, thoughtful, and attentive to others, Tom focused on "the mistake" he had made. He shared how embarrassed he was. What would others think of him? Tom never gave many details. I never really found out how Tom developed AIDS.

Tom worried about his friends from whom he had pulled away. So many unanswered telephone calls and notes! He admitted that he had protected himself and withdrawn. He went through periods of shame. At times, despair was his only companion. He shared the loneliness that all of this created for him.

One day, Tom asked me to contact his friend Anna and ask if she would like to visit him. Tom and Anna had been very good friends but had not seen each other in over two years. He was too ashamed to tell her about his condition.

When I spoke with Anna, the betrayal and abandonment that Anna felt was evidenced in her words. "Why didn't he tell me what was going on?" she cried. I wasn't sure if Anna would even go to visit Tom.

The next morning Anna called me and asked what time visiting hours were at the hospital. I agreed to take her over when I went for my visit. When we walked into the room, both old friends seemed very frightened of each other. But when they embraced, the conversation immediately came more easily.

"What did I ever do that you cut me off?" Anna asked.

"You didn't do a thing. I was so ashamed to tell you about myself."

"It doesn't matter to me. I've missed you and have worried about you so."

"Anna, I'm glad you came. I'm so sorry. Please forgive me."

Tears flowed. Two friends were reunited.

One of Tom's last conversations was with his brother. Tom told him, "I do have AIDS. But I know I am a good person, and I hope you love me."

Tom's brother went over to his brother's bedside and embraced him. "Yes I love you. I love you so much. I don't care what you have. I love you."

Tom's father still remained distant, but it seemed to me that even he and Tom had somewhat repaired their rift by the time of Tom's death. The night of Tom's wake, his father embraced me and said, "I wanted a perfect son. For a while I thought he was a failure. But these weeks in the hospital I started to learn who my son was again. I loved him so much. He was a good boy. I am proud of my son."

Tom had died knowing that his father accepted and loved him and that even when we make mistakes we can be perfect.

FALL SEVEN TIMES,
STAND UP EIGHT.

Japanese Proverb

WAY 2 :

Change Your Self-Talk

The running conversation we carry on in our head is endless. We are always thinking and rethinking. A continuous stream of messages comes to us. When the messages are negative, then we tend to internalize the negativity. A self-fulfilling prophecy arises; for example, when we tell ourselves we can't do something, inevitably we can't.

Our self-talk can become the script whereby we live our lives. Our fears, our doubts, our self-defeating scripts can take center stage. Self-talk has lots of power! But, we can change our negative self-talk. And, if we wish to reduce our stress levels, changing our self-talk becomes essential.

The grade school I attended was in a safe and secure little city where everyone knew and cared for each other. People respected other people's property, and expressions of thoughtfulness to neighbors were common. I attended a parochial grade school that was only a half block from my house. The neighborhood felt like one big family.

When I was in the third grade I had a wonderful teacher who brought the best out of each student. She made school fun, which motivated us to strive for good grades, study hard, and really learn all we could. When the report cards were given out all the kids would compare their marks. Each of us wanted to have the highest average.

The last report card in June was an important one because our final grades gave status as we entered the next grade. I still remember looking at my final average of 99.4. I was thrilled. And then I found out that my classmate Jimmy had a 99.6. Two-tenths of a point higher than mine! It came down to Jimmy spelling one word that I couldn't spell. On that day, I decided once and for all that I couldn't spell. As I carried that self-defeating message around in my head, it evolved into truth, a truth that has taken a long time to dispel.

We must be careful what we tell ourselves. An incident in the life of author Norman Cousins points this out. Cousins was scheduled to give several lectures. He was feeling exhausted and needed a break. Looking at his calendar, he realized that he was scheduled to speak every day for the next two weeks. Some of those days he was to give two lectures. Cousins asked his secretary to cancel out his next two days. He admitted to her that he was exhausted and needed a break. She told him he could not just cancel out like that.

"What do you mean I can't do that?" he asked.

His devoted secretary responded that it wasn't like he just had a heart attack. Cousins acquiesced. She was right, he told himself.

Well, two years later Norman Cousins did have a heart attack. Now in his mind he had earned the right to cancel out his calendar and to rest. Like the case of Cousins, the messages we speak in our minds often become actualized.

If we tell ourselves we can't spell or we are dumb or we're incapable of learning how to use a computer, then we internalize those messages until those things actually become true. Our self-talk begins to give definition to our self-esteem. We begin to become who we tell ourselves we are.

Negative and critical self-talk feeds our stress level. The good news is that we do have the power to change negative self-talk into positive self-talk. We do this whenever we empower ourselves with beliefs and understanding that help us acknowledge our goodness and the positive strengths with which we have been blessed. Our stress level is decreased when our self-talk is positive.

We can change our self-talk from positive to negative by listening more carefully to what we are saying to ourselves about a situation or frustration. Just telling ourselves that we can change sets the process in motion.

WITH OUR THOUGHTS WE MAKE OUR WORLD. THINK EVIL THOUGHTS AND EVIL WILL FOLLOW YOU AS SURELY AS THE CART FOLLOWS THE OX.

Siddhartha Gautama

Change Your Self-Talk

- Listen to your thoughts and hear whether they are negative or positive. If your messages are only negative, then nothing will be right. If your messages are positive, you perceive situations positively. Once you become aware of your negative self-talk you can change it. So spend some time listening to what you are saying to yourself. Keep a log of your self-talk if you find that helpful.

- One way of transforming our self-talk is by reciting a single, positive word or affirming phrase in harmony with our breathing. Deep breathing on its own can help us reduce stress and feel more balanced; adding the message of a positive word or phrase plants positive self-talk in our spirit. This form of breathing with an empowering word or phrase is common to most of the world's great religions. Its Christian formulation can be found in a book called *The Cloud of Unknowing* by an anonymous English priest of the fourteenth century. He explains breathing with a word this way:

  > If you want to gather all your desire into one simple word that the mind can easily retain, choose a short word rather than a long one. A one-syllable word such as "God" or "love" is best. But choose one that is meaningful to you. Then fix it in your mind so that it will remain there come what may. This word will be your defense in conflict and in peace. Use it to beat upon the cloud of darkness about you and to subdue all distractions.

  > Repeating the single word or short phrase can be powerful. Here are steps to follow: First, sit relaxed. Still yourself by stretching and deep

breathing. Then choose a single word or short phrase that somehow expresses your deepest values and is empowering. It might be a name of God (e.g., Wisdom, Allah, Light) or another soothing, centering word or phrase: peace, love, goodness, hope, calm. Begin repeating this word phrase inwardly in harmony with your breathing. If your mind wanders or you get distracted, gently start repeating your word again. End with some expression of gratitude: a prayer of thanks, a smile. This form of centered breathing can be done anywhere and any time that you need positive self-talk.

- Think about what is bothering you. It can be a family problem, an upcoming social event, a work-related issue, or a lingering hurt with a significant person. Is there something you can do about it? Think about people you could go to and ask for help or for advice. Work out a plan to address the problem. Then you are in charge. Do not let your negative self-talk go unanswered.

- Make a list of several positive messages that you need to tell yourself every day. For example, "I can keep confidences" or "I am dependable." Read through the list—several times a day if necessary— and engage in some positive self-talk until you truly believe each message.

WHAT LIES BEHIND US AND WHAT LIES BEFORE US ARE TINY MATTERS COMPARED TO WHAT LIES WITHIN US.

Ralph Waldo Emerson

A Conversation of Sorts

I'm talking to myself all day. Now before you wonder about my sanity, I think I'm pretty normal in sending messages to myself that do seem to affect the way I interact with the world. The messages that I send can be encouraging, supportive, and nurturing. However, I can also send messages that could be destructive of or harmful to my self-esteem. When I am bombarded with the inevitable stressors throughout the day, what I'm saying to myself influences how effectively I handle daily situations. More important, my words can affect my inner peace.

As a management consultant and trainer, I encourage clients in coaching situations to become aware of the messages they are sending themselves. Are these messages positive or negative? Do they motivate or discourage? I try to share with my clients what I have learned over the years that has been helpful to me.

Several years ago, I was providing skills training for a manufacturing group. Management had reorganized line employees into teams, which meant that many of the employees had to learn new skills after doing the same job for fifteen to twenty years. The older women and men were grouped with younger, more adaptable folks who often were impatient with the amount of time it took for their older co-workers to learn a new task.

Management had hired me to teach the employees better communication skills and to provide team-building experiences. I worked with six different teams. An older woman on one team persistently looked anxious and tense. Sarah seemed to be willing herself to understand the processes I was teaching. The fearful look on her face told me that she wasn't experiencing success in grasping the concepts. Finally, practically in tears, she came to me after a particularly difficult session on offering constructive feedback.

"I'm never going to be able to make the change. I can't learn the new job, and the others are so much faster than me."

At forty-five, she felt too old and feared that she was going to lose her job. In addition, she just couldn't get along with her other teammates because she thought they all hated her. She tried to be friends. She even bought them gifts. But she just didn't feel good enough. The stress at work had started taking its toll on her home life.

After listening to Sarah's litany of fears, I asked her what she thought of the messages she was giving herself. All I heard was that she was "too old, too unlikable, and too slow." We talked about her work before the change. How did she do? Was she successful? Did she make her goal each week?

"I always made my goal. Not much over, but I did good enough. But these young girls can go so much faster than I can."

We talked about her accomplishments as a wife and mother, and she described how she was able to keep house, raise kids, work all these years, and handle all of these responsibilities fairly effectively. Her face began to brighten as she realized that she had been successful in many areas of her life.

"Now let's take a look at those messages you've been giving yourself," I directed. "See if you can turn them around to positive statements."

"You mean the one about my being too old?" she asked before continuing. "I have experience, a lot more than those young girls. I am an experienced worker."

"Good," I responded. "Now what about this idea that you can't learn new things? Didn't you tell me that a few years ago you set up a new workflow process over in assembly? You can't have changed that much over five years."

"I guess I can try to learn the new ways. It just seems too much at one time."

"So break it down into smaller parts. And remember all the times you've been successful in the past."

I encouraged her to tell herself during the following two weeks between classes that she was a competent employee who was capable of learning new skills. Because of her years of experience, she was able to thoughtfully analyze a problem and figure out a way to make the new position work. She wrote out two affirmations that she was going to read every day before work. She planned to keep them in her pocket and refer to them throughout the day.

Two weeks later I returned to the plant for the next session. Before the other employees arrived, Sarah came in with a gleam in her eye.

"It works," she exclaimed. "Well, almost, anyway. I said the affirmations every day. I still am having problems with speed, but I finally know how to run the cutter. But best of all, I'm not as afraid as before."

Sarah went on to explain that she wasn't as nervous about coming to work. Except for a couple of days the previous week, which were terrors, she went home less upset.

After the session that day, we worked on two more affirmations that she could use. I met with Sarah four more times after that. Each time she seemed to feel more confident. This new strength didn't come easily to her, and she often stumbled. But she was determined not to let all those negative messages keep her from at least trying to succeed. She had burdened herself with such negative self-talk that she never felt good about herself. This added stress to an already stressful day.

About a year later, I ran into Sarah at the grocery store. She greeted me like a long-lost friend and told me that she was doing okay. Sarah felt fine about never becoming a superstar, but rather handling the job well enough. She was particularly happy that she was not afraid as much as she used to be.

"Whenever the stress starts to build up, I just pull out my messages, start talking to myself, and things get back on track. I can do it. I am doing it."

Rosalie Hooper-Thomas

NOTHING ERASES UNPLEASANT THOUGHTS MORE EFFECTIVELY THAN CONCENTRATION ON PLEASANT ONES.

Hans Selye

Book Signing

One of the most touching notes I have ever received came to me two days after a book signing that I did at a Barnes and Noble.

When I do book signings, I usually give a half-hour talk as part of the event. Arriving that day at the bookstore about seven minutes early, I found all the chairs that had been set up were filled. People were sitting on the windowsills. The standing crowd seemed to be growing. I was exhilarated by the number of people. As with most lecturers, my audience energizes me, and looking at their faces indicates to me how I am doing.

I was thoroughly enjoying myself, talking about humor and the benefits one gets from humor. Laughter is such a wonderful connector, and I was "connecting" with this group. Their laughter was a gift back to me. I usually ask people to be good to themselves and to learn to relax a bit.

After about a half-hour of the talk, I got down to the business of signing books. I always try to engage in a short conversation with the person for whom I am signing a book. I trust myself to say what comes into my mind at that time. Sometimes it is in reference to what the person is telling me. Sometimes it has to do with a remark or an expression that person had on their face during my presentation.

The note I received after this event began by thanking me for sharing my sense of humor. A few sentences into the note I read: "There were so many people for your signing, and I doubt you will remember me—second row by the window with a blue vest—but you made a comment to me that I was making eye contact with you and had a great, warm smile."

I did remember the woman. As the note continued, she told me how much the comment meant to her. She then shared her story with me. It seems we had crossed paths before. She told me that five years before she had come to our counseling center during a difficult time in her life. After her session, she sat waiting for her husband to come and pick her up. She remembered that each time I walked past the doorway I would smile at her. Unfortunately, the woman's condition required hospitalization.

Then she wrote, "Just three months ago I doused myself with gasoline and was going to set myself afire—the ultimate sacrifice to God for my many sins." She continued, "I now thank God that my husband found me before it was too late."

The woman said that she was still seeing a psychiatrist twice weekly and had "made incredible progress, but eye contact and humor don't come easily. When you made note of it to me, all I could think of was 'Wow. Me? Incredible!'"

She closed by thanking me for "words that meant so much."

I thanked her for the note, and realized once again that we never know how our words affect another person. We are not aware of the impact we have. We never know what people are carrying in their hearts.

Her self-talk had led her to the brink of self-destruction. My talk had helped her back. Now she had begun the long road back to health by talking to herself in new and positive ways. What a privilege for me to have received this note and shared her story.

THE MIND IS ITS OWN PLACE AND IN ITSELF CAN MAKE A HEAVEN OF HELL, A HELL OF HEAVEN.

John Milton

WAY 3 :

Prioritize

I MUST GOVERN THE CLOCK, NOT
BE GOVERNED BY IT.

Golda Meir

Busy is definitely the name of the game today. For
example, parents recite lists with a million things
they must do each day, leaving themselves no free time.
They are taxi drivers for their children to their sporting
events, dance classes, and music lessons. Parents also
have to monitor homework and make time for church
commitments. In between all of the extracurricular
activities, parents must find time to go to work, prepare
meals, clean the house, do the laundry—besides doing
volunteer work, maintaining extended family relationships, and sleeping. Sleep comes more from
exhaustion.

It would be wise for us to remember that all living
persons have the same number of seconds in each day
(86,400). No one is given one second more or less. Yet,
we can all choose to use our time each day in whatever
way we choose. It is how we prioritize its use and how

we choose to spend it that can help us bring quality to our lives.

There is an old story about three masons who are laying bricks. A man walks up to them and asks them each the same question: "What are you doing?" The first mason spits on the ground and looks up. "I'm laying bricks. What does it look like I'm doing?" The second mason groans and mops his brow. "I'm earning a living." The third mason looks up with light in his eyes and says, "I'm building a cathedral." Who do you think feels most refreshed at the end of the day? Whose perspective is most positive and rewarding?

Similarly, a maxim from the east teaches that "thoughts are things." Our attitudes and perceptions determine how we prioritize our life. In order to keep our day balanced and wholesome, we must take charge of our decisions about time and determine what is important. We cannot enjoy a friend's presence if we are feeling frazzled, fragmented, or pulled from every side. We cannot see the gifts and blessings in front of us if we are looking down the road at the next crisis that might occur. We cannot see the "cathedral" if we concentrate on the "bricks" or "paycheck."

We need to begin asking, "What really matters?" Our lives might be lived quite differently if we asked this question more often. Perhaps we would choose to fly a kite with our child instead of working overtime, go to a movie with a friend, sit still in the backyard and look at the beauty of the sky at dusk, see the face of God in a newborn baby, feel the blessings given to us by an older person as we sit and listen to a story they love to tell over and over again.

This brings to mind the story told of a woman who longed to find out what heaven was like. She prayed constantly for this knowledge. One night she had a dream. In the dream an angel came and took her to heaven. They walked down a street and when they came to an ordinary looking house, the angel said, "Go and look inside."

So the woman walked into the house and there she found a woman preparing dinner, another person reading the paper, and children playing games. The woman turned to the angel and asked, "Is this all there is to heaven?"

The angel replied, "Those people you saw in the house are not in paradise. Paradise is in them."

At the end of our life will we really care about all the hours we worked, all the committees we sat on, or even all the money we accumulated? Or will we wish we had spent more time laughing, talking to loved ones, relaxing, and filling our hearts and souls with life-giving memories? My guess is that we would choose the latter.

If we prioritize our day and keep what is important as our focus, we will enjoy life more and decrease our stress. We won't feel guilty when we take those moments with our loved ones and take the time to do the things we really enjoy doing, just for the sake of doing them.

Learning to relax is not a lesson our culture teaches us. Unwinding is hard to do. We need to practice prioritizing, separating the important from the unimportant. Relaxing a bit and setting priorities reduce stress in our lives because these skills give us time to find the paradise that is inside us right now.

> IF WE WANT TO BREAK OUT OF THE
> MECHANISTIC AND OBSESSIVE SORT
> OF ACTION . . . WE MUST FIRST
> LEARN TO ASK OURSELVES A SIMPLE
> QUESTION: "WHY AM I DOING
> THIS?"
>
> *Parker Palmer*

Prioritize

- If you had only six months to live, how would you spend your time? Write your thoughts in a journal, for example:
  - Who would you want to spend the most time with?
  - What would you want to be sure you did?
  - What do you find the best part of living?
- Write three values you hold that are most important to you.
  - Now number them 1, 2, and 3 in order of importance to you.
  - If someone audited your daily schedule, how would these values be manifest in the way you spent your time?
- Make a list of dreams you want to accomplish in your life. After each dream, write what you would

have to do in order to make your dream come true. Be realistic. Everything cannot be accomplished in a day or a week.

- Take your calendar and mark at least two times per month for you to do something for yourself (for example, going to a movie or out to dinner).

- Set your boundaries. Considering your answers to the first three exercises—what you would do if you had only a year to live, your three most important values, and the list of your dreams—set some boundaries on those actions that regularly interfere with you following your priorities. For example: Value—spending time on weekends with my spouse and children. Boundary—I will not check my office e-mails on weekends or do office work on Sundays. Set some boundary on several actions that get in the way of achieving your priorities, including your dreams.

- Get up right now and do something completely "useless" but that fits in with your values and priorities like: hugging a loved one, listening to a favorite CD, baking cookies, shooting baskets with your teenager, whistling while walking around the block with your dog, planting some flower bulbs, or making a snow angel.

- One way of keeping track of your priorities is to keep a daily journal. In her book *Life's Companion*, Christina Baldwin says that, "Flow writing reveals the mind's agenda underneath the busyness of surface thoughts." This is a particularly useful method for letting out what is stressing us and, when we are finished, realizing if our actions that day forwarded our purpose in life. Directions: Put pen to paper and begin writing. Maybe write about whatever happened during the day. Write about someone you met. However, do not bother to formulate thoughts; just let what comes out, come out. Keep the pen moving. If you get stuck, write down names of objects in the room, and then keep going. When you feel written out, just stop. Note any feelings about how the day matched your priorities.

ONE WAY TO GET HIGH BLOOD PRESSURE IS TO GO MOUNTAIN CLIMBING OVER MOLEHILLS.

Earl Wilson

Important Things First

Steve and Joan, a couple who had been married for five years, decided they needed a marriage counselor. Steve was a machine-shop operator who worked long hours to pay for all the family's expenses. Joan stayed home with their two children, ages one and two.

Steve would come home from work and never get past the kitchen. It was a mess. Dishes in the sink. Cereal on the floor. Toys all over. Steve and Joan long ago agreed that cooking supper was his responsibility, but before he could even begin cooking he would have to clean.

Joan was overwhelmed with the demands of two babies. Never was there one moment of peace and quiet.

By the time the children were fed, given baths, and put in their cribs it was at least eight o'clock. Then Steve and Joan would sit down to their suppers. Steve liked to watch television while they ate. When he would finish he would go into the den where he would watch more TV. This put Joan at her wits' end: "How can he sit there and watch a football game? I'm exhausted. He hasn't said anything to me except the kitchen is a mess again."

Night after night the scene replayed itself. They came to counseling because they both realized that there had to be more to life than this type of existence.

The first session was filled with each describing the other's behaviors. Joan's version said: All Steve does is go to work, come home, clean the kitchen, yell about the kids making too much noise, and watch television. Steve wondered what Joan did all day long. She didn't work, the kids took naps, and the house was always a mess. Both found themselves curt in responding to the other.

A solution was offered: What twenty minutes a day could be theirs with no children and no television? Just twenty minutes to talk to and be with each other.

It seemed impossible for them to decide. Television relaxed Steve, he said. Steve worked six days a week and likes to play golf on his day off. (Joan wondered when she got a day off.)

Several sessions later both began to realize what they wanted their life to look like. They wanted a happy marriage. They wanted healthy, happy children. They wanted a solid family life. The television in the kitchen was the first thing to go. Suppertime would be a time for conversation. It turns out that after supper they would even find themselves sitting next to each other on the couch and snuggling for a few extra minutes.

Steve also decided he didn't need to play golf every week. And when he did play, he agreed to play nine holes instead of eighteen. That would give him more family time.

Joan decided to lighten up on conversations, not to always be preaching to Steve and correcting him. She also decided she would keep the kitchen clean, get supper started, so that it would give them a bit more relaxing time together.

Setting priorities helped them decide what was important. They then had a framework to make these things happen, and it slowly removed much of the stress that threatened their marriage.

FINISH EACH DAY AND BE DONE

WITH IT.

YOU HAVE DONE WHAT YOU COULD;

SOME BLUNDERS AND ABSURDITIES

NO DOUBT CREPT IN.

FORGET THEM AS SOON AS YOU CAN.

TOMORROW IS A NEW DAY,

YOU SHALL BEGIN IT WELL AND

SERENELY.

Ralph Waldo Emerson

Two Left Shoes

E ach day of life has incomparable value. As we begin to realize that we don't know how many of those precious days we have, we begin to shift our priorities.

I remember being invited to Utica to address a conference. The drive between Albany and Utica, New York, usually takes about an hour and a half. When I awoke that morning, I looked out my bedroom window to see that we had been gifted with eight inches of snow overnight. The snow continued to come down.

Even so, my goal was to get to Utica on time. I dressed frantically, grabbed what I needed, hurried out of the house, and threw my briefcase in my car.

Driving was treacherous. Snow covered the streets, and visibility was limited. With nothing else that I could do, I held on tight to the steering wheel, stayed very attentive, and prayed.

I arrived at the convention address about five minutes late. Considering the weather conditions, I had done exceedingly well. I jumped out of the car and grabbed my briefcase and my shoes. Because of the amount of snow I had worn boots. My intent was to change them when I got into the auditorium.

The person at the podium saw me come into the back of the auditorium. She announced that I had arrived, and we could begin. As she was reading my introduction and giving my background to the participants, I removed my winter coat and boots. Reaching into my bag, I first pulled out a blue shoe and then a black shoe. Then I rudely discovered that besides being different colors they were both left shoes! In a quandary, I stood looking at the shoes. No way could I get my right foot in my left shoe.

Just as I was staring at my two left shoes, the woman giving the introduction was saying, "And we are so pleased to have Anne Bryan Smollin with us this morning to help us get started on the right foot."

I walked out on the stage in my stocking feet, carrying my two left shoes. I had to decide what was important, my appearance or the content of my message. Needless to say, it was a great opening for me. I suppose I had my priorities straight. Giving the conference to a welcoming audience, sharing what I had learned, and arriving safely were more important than having the right shoes. Besides, we all got a laugh out of the story, and that's always a good way to begin a conversation or presentation.

Illness helps us to put a premium on what is really important, and what is not. My friend Rose Ann who has ALS, or Lou Gehrig's disease, wrote me a note regarding her birthday celebration: "I used to think, 'O God, another birthday!' and now I say 'Thank God, another birthday!'" People and life-giving moments become newly important. Dean Ornish remarked, "Love and intimacy are at the root of what makes us sick and what makes us well, what causes sadness and what bring happiness, what makes us suffer and what leads to healing." How often we've heard people remind us that we don't appreciate our good health until we become ill. We value proving our mettle and sticking to time schedules, as opposed to paying attention to our immediate tasks. I'm afraid that most of us are slow learners, myself included. Except on the day when I had only two left shoes.

SLOW DOWN AND ENJOY LIFE. IT'S
NOT ONLY THE SCENERY YOU MISS
BY GOING TOO FAST—YOU ALSO
MISS THE SENSE OF WHERE YOU ARE
GOING AND WHY.

Eddie Cantor

WAY 4 :

Be Present Where You Are

SANITY PROCLAIMS THAT IMMEDIATE
AWARENESS IS SIMPLY A STATE OF
APPRECIATION. ONE NEED DO
NOTHING, NOTHING AT ALL WITH IT.

Gerald May

There is a wonderful Zen story that reminds us to be present where we are and to be open to the truth that is in front of us. It goes like this:

A young widower returned home one day to find his house burned down and his five-year-old son lost. Near the ruins of his house was the charred corpse of a child. The widower wept and wept and wept. After the child's cremation, he kept the ashes in a bag and carried them with him day and night.

But his son had not perished in the fire. Bandits had taken him off. One day the boy escaped and returned to his father's house. The son arrived at midnight and knocked at the door. "Who are you?" asked the father. "I am your son."

"You are lying. My son died more than three months ago."

The father persisted in his unbelief and would not open the door. After a while the son left and the father lost his son forever.

So often we cannot live in the now, cannot accept the truth that knocks at the door in the present moment. Some live in yesterday. "If only I had said this. . . . If only I had done that. . . . "

Well, we can't change yesterday. We have no control over it. We can't take a word back that we said or redo a thing we did. The past is gone. There is no power in yesterday unless we hold on to it. In the same way, tomorrow has power over us only if we worry about it. We can all hope for tomorrow, but none of us is truly assured of it.

What we do have is the present moment. This is the moment that contains all that we need. It has energy and humor and the grace needed to move into the next moment. Slowing down to live this present moment is not always easy.

To live in the present takes trust. We have to believe that this moment is where the energy source is. If we need to be in control of everything, then most likely we are always living in the future. Thus, we plan, organize, and orchestrate so that things happen the way we want them to. But the problem is that we have missed this moment.

Living the moment opens our world to the surprises and the wonders of that moment. Enjoy one breath at a time. Really see the wonder of creation. Be touched by a friend's warm smile. Savor this moment, then the next, and the next. Each in turn, each alone. One doesn't make the grass grow, as the Chinese saying goes, by pulling it. It grows as it will, moment by moment.

In the Broadway musical *The Music Man*, the flamboyant salesman, Professor Harold Hill, attempts to get Marian, the librarian, to go on a date with him. Professor Hill asks Marian to meet him by the footbridge of a stream in the city park. Marian wants to go but is fearful, so she refuses, saying, "Please, some other time. Maybe tomorrow."

The ever-persistent salesman, Hill continues to tempt her to meet him at the bridge, but she continually finds excuses to postpone the date. In exasperation, he utters those marvelous words well worth remembering, "Pile up enough tomorrows, and you'll find you have collected nothing but a lot of empty yesterdays."

We need to live the moment. Seize the present moment and choose the life in it. Notice everything and everyone around us. Be kind to those who are near. If this were our last minute on earth would we want it spent being angry over a traffic jam or appreciating the beauty in front of us? Just think about the people on the Titanic who passed up dessert!

Laughter is one way of staying present to the moment. Laughter reduces the stress and gives us the ability to handle the hard moments. Laughter creates a bond and helps us deal constructively with the moment. Laughter is a blessing, and it touches the soul of each person. It doesn't let us race ahead or stay stuck in the past.

Living in the present and experiencing the present moment is a gift we give to ourselves. There is a wonderful story of a Japanese general who was arrested by the enemy and thrown into prison. He knew that the next day he was going to be tortured. He tossed and turned all night in his prison cell, unable to sleep. Then the realization struck him: "When am I going to

be tortured? Tomorrow? But tomorrow is not real—
that's what my Zen master taught me." The moment
he realized this he calmed down and fell asleep. He
realized that the only thing is now. Even though he
was in prison, he was a free man.

The enemies to freedom are not outside of us but
within us. As Ralph Waldo Emerson pointed out,
"What lies behind us and what lies before us are tiny
matters compared to what lies within us." The present
moment can be taken in and savored. It is real.

Nothing is worth more than
this day.

Goethe

Be Present Where You Are

- Stop all your activity right now. Just sit still. Take
  time to look at what's going on around you. What
  do you see? What do you hear? What do you feel?
  Being attentive and aware of the moment helps you
  to be aware of what you are doing. You live the one
  precious moment in front of you.

- Take a deep breath. Now slowly exhale. Repeat this
  five times. Feel your body relax. Feel the present
  moment.

- Let go of the past. Don't drain yourself by holding on to yesterday. It has no power. Now is what is important. This very minute. This very second. If letting go is a problem, here is an exercise that might help:

  > Sit quietly with your eyes closed. Rest your hands on your lap with your palms facing down. Invite all the worries and concerns about the past to flood into your mind. As each worry starts to pull you into its grip, let go of it. Imagine that you are dropping it out of the palm of your hand into the vastness of space or into the hand of God. Drop each source of worry and concern. Let them all go; give them away. Then, when you have released them all, turn your hands palms up. Now invite the present in. Ask the gift of the present into your life. Just be aware of this present moment. When you have quieted and relaxed, give thanks for the gift of the present moment.

- Make time to be with a friend. If you can't find the time for dinner, then make a phone call. Send a joke by e-mail or postcard. You will get more from that simple gift than the one who receives it.

- Go outside and walk around the block or through a park. As you go along, notice what is around you. Just look, listen, feel, and smell. Celebrate sensation. If you start thinking about something—your next project, a worry, some decision—gently refocus back on whatever is right in front of you. If it helps, simply tell yourself, "I am walking now" or "I am watching the clouds pass overhead." Engage the present moment.

AS YOU WALK, EAT, AND TRAVEL, BE
WHERE YOU ARE. OTHERWISE, YOU
WILL MISS YOUR LIFE.

Siddhartha Gautama

Rose Ann

Rose Ann and I have been friends for years. I've watched her children grow up, and I've gotten them out of more jams than she will ever know. I would vacation the first week of August every year with the family. She has been my friend in the truest sense of the word for years. We've laughed together, cried together, given up candy for Lent together, shared diets—you know, all the things that really bond two people together.

About a year and a half ago, Rose Ann was diagnosed with ALS (more commonly known as Lou Gehrig's disease). She now lives about four and a half hours away, and I try to get to see her as often as possible. One time, driving down to her home, I found myself preparing for whom I would see. It was evident from our phone calls that she was having a hard time speaking. She had lost the ability to walk and now had an electric wheelchair, a fire engine red one. Rose Ann told me on the phone, "If I'm going, I'm going out in style." Rose Ann also has a trained dog named Bear that is her guide and protector.

I didn't want to change my expression when I walked into her home. That is not easy with friends. She knew me well and knew that I wear my feelings on my face and that they are reflected in my eyes. I just wanted to protect her—or maybe I wanted to protect myself. After all, this was my friend.

I walked into her house, and she was anxiously awaiting my visit. She looked at me and said, "Don't kiss me. I have diarrhea, and I don't want you to get it."

I instantly replied, "Oh, so that's how you get it. I've always wondered." Everyone in the room burst out laughing. Thank God.

My worries over how I would act vanished into the pleasure of the present moment.

IN ETERNITY THERE IS INDEED SOMETHING TRUE AND SUBLIME. BUT ALL THESE TIMES AND PLACES AND OCCASIONS ARE NOW AND HERE. GOD CULMINATES IN THE PRESENT MOMENT, AND WILL NEVER BE MORE DIVINE IN THE LAPSE OF ALL THE AGES.

Henry David Thoreau

Stars in the Driveway

A friend told me this story about enjoying the present moment:

Jo's late night phone call surprised me. She had not called or returned one of my voice-mail messages in weeks. Undoubtedly something was up. "Joyce," she sobbed, "I've got to talk to you. I know I've been distant, but I really need your help now. Can you come over?"

"Okay. Have tea ready. Sounds like we're gonna need it."

Jo and I had been college roommates. Contrary to what usually happens to roommates, we became fast friends. We were one another's bridesmaids, had kids close in age and, while she was still married, we did things together and with our families. Eighteen months ago, Jo's husband, Aaron, had announced that he wanted out of the marriage. Unbeknownst to Jo, he had taken a job in Minnesota. He planned to move in three weeks. "Now I'll get my chance in life. You've had yours," he concluded.

Jo and Aaron had been arguing more often, but the announcement caught Jo off balance. She knew that Aaron resented her larger paycheck, her circle of friends, and when she could admit it, her competence. Jo loved nursing. She hated the paperwork and the increasing bureaucracy, but she learned to manage it. Over several years, she had finished training to be a nurse practitioner. Her patients loved her, and the clinic kept raising her salary. She was also the one whom organizations often tapped to chair fund drives or to give talks. When she had to be gone in the evenings,

Aaron declared that he would stay at home with their two children, but the declaration had gradually turned into a surly accusation. Eventually, mere irritants became major issues. Now he was gone.

As I pulled into Jo's driveway, I saw the kitchen lights on. I didn't have to knock. Jo flung open the back door and, sobbing, fell into my arms.

"Joyce, I'm such a failure. Oh, God, Aaron's a pig. I can't go on this way. I almost slapped Timmy tonight."

I got her seated and poured us both some tea. "You better start from the beginning. Get me up to speed."

"Joyce, it's gotten bad. I'm at the end of my rope. Tonight I picked up the kids at daycare, late as usual. They were whiny about it. It was the fifth day in a row, but things at the clinic have been crazy too." Jo had arrived at home with the kids still complaining, then fussing with each other. Frazzled from work and the kids, she walked into a scene of destruction. Their calico cat, Sophie, stretched out on top of the refrigerator, yawned, ignoring the mess she had made. Somehow in her journey across the kitchen counters and appliances, she had knocked the Friar Tuck cookie jar off the counter, shattering it into a million shards. Pasta shells were scattered amidst splinters of glass from the decanter that Sophie had displaced from its perch over the stove.

"I grabbed Sophie off the fridge. She got scared and scratched the hell out of me. I got even angrier and threw her out the back door. Then Timmy yelled that I hurt Sophie and started crying. I had my hand up to slap him and caught myself just in time. Then Pam joined in. I yelled for them to go to their rooms, change clothes, and get ready for supper, and stop whining. Neither of them ate much. When I told the kids to get ready for bed, for once they didn't argue. When I came in to read to them—a sacred custom—both Timmy and Pam pretended to sleep.

"Joyce, I came into the kitchen after they fell asleep and just broke down. I had forgotten about poor Sophie too. Poor girl scratched on the door. When I let her in she ran into the living room instead of curling around my leg. That's when I called you."

Jo started weeping again. "What am I gonna do?"

We talked long through the night. Jo needed that. She had been the one everyone depended on for so long that she had forgotten how to ask for help herself. When I left, we hugged deeply. As she walked me out to the car, just as I was getting in, she stopped me. Staring up into the starry sky, she said, "Joyce, look, there's the Big Dipper. I haven't seen it in a long time. But then," she paused, "I haven't seen a lot of things since Aaron left. Maybe things will be better if I start seeing good stuff again." I hope so, dear Jo, I thought as I backed out of the driveway.

Jo and I are closer than ever now. She dropped off a couple of committees and pulled out of her church choir. Instead of frantic phone calls now, I get messages like the one I had last Saturday afternoon. "Joycie, get your kids in the car. Let's drive up to Wildcat Mountain State Park and look at the fall colors. Have you been noticing how the ash leaves are almost gone, while the silver maples are just turning?" So we went.

While the kids were running around in the woods, Jo and I sat on the overlook. I asked, "How you doing?"

Smiling, Jo hugged me around the shoulder. "I'm good. Honestly. Thank you, Joycie. You saved my fanny that night. So did the stars. I know it sounds weird, but it hit me right there in the driveway that I'd been miss-ing all the good things—the little things. I got so wrapped up in my anger at Aaron, the frantic pace at work, and this tremendous feeling of responsibility for the kids that I hadn't paid attention to anyone or anything right in front of me. After you left, I went into the kids' room. They were so precious, so beautiful sleeping there. It took my breath away. I swore to myself that I had to let go of Aaron and start living right then. Life's too damned short to let it slip away. Now, come on, let's get the grill going and help the kids burn some wieners."

IF YOU PAY ATTENTION, WISDOM WILL BE YOURS.

Book of Ecclesiasticus

WAY 5 :

Avoid Crazymakers

IN EACH HUMAN HEART ARE A
TIGER, A PIG, AN ASS AND A
NIGHTINGALE. DIVERSITY OF CHAR-
ACTER IS DUE TO THEIR UNEQUAL
ACTIVITY.

Ambrose Bierce

Some people just know how to press our buttons. They have the secret code to raising our blood pressure and frustrating us beyond words. They drain our energy and anxiety marches in at the very sound of their names. These people always reverse everything so it is your fault and not theirs. They are masters of blame. They are continually late for meetings and appointments and are always busier and more important than anyone else. They withhold information from others because, to them, information is power. They are the people who give you a gift and expect you to use it immediately and in the way that they would use it. They are the persons who set a lunch date with you and then have to cancel because they forgot to put it in their calendar or because something better came along. They are people who have unrealistic expectations of us. They are the people who live the Yiddish proverb: "Sleep faster . . . We need the pillows!"

Just hearing the name of one of these crazymakers—and we all know people like these—causes stress in our lives. They are a drag to be around. They make our bodies tighten, our muscles tense up. We dread their appearance or hearing their voices on the other end of the phone.

Toxic people drain our energy. Crazymakers like these may sometimes be categorized as pessimists, complainers, ingrates, and manipulators. They are most always negative. They think the world owes them a living.

Crazymakers are often people who are charismatic and highly persuasive. They expect special treatment, have no boundaries, and never respect the boundaries of others. If we are not careful, they can take over our whole life.

But these people have power over us only if we give to it them. For us to be healthy, it is better not to spend a lot of time with or concerning ourselves over crazymakers lest we internalize their negativity. There is no reason for us to be around so much chaos and negativity.

On the other hand, some wonderful people come into our lives and leave their marks on our hearts and souls. Eddie Pu, a national park ranger in Hawaii, was once such man. Eddie is a man of integrity and wisdom. He is a person everyone wants to be around. And Eddie is always smiling. Once I asked Eddie why he smiled so much. He looked puzzled and said, "I don't know that I am. When the wind blows, the leaves are waving—they're smiling. When you throw a rock into a pool and ripples go out—the water is smiling. That's the energy. That's what I call my energy." This is energy that brings us life.

We are never the same again after meeting life-givers like Eddie Pu. These people are positive, healthy, and holy people who give energy to others. They encourage us to keep going. They praise and affirm our efforts and our successes. They help us believe in ourselves and know who God truly is. We can never truly know God unless we see the reflection of God in the eyes of another. We need our hearts to be touched by people who believe in themselves and live life fully each moment.

We can't change anyone else. We have no control over the way other people behave. People act the way they want to act, not the way we want them to act. We can only change ourselves. The point of this chapter is to remind you to recognize and avoid the crazymakers and embrace life-givers in your life if you want a less stressful and more harmonious life.

WORRY IS LIKE BLOOD PRESSURE:
YOU NEED A CERTAIN LEVEL TO
LIVE, BUT TOO MUCH CAN KILL YOU.

Edward M. Hallowell

Avoid Crazymakers

- List the names of ten friends, both old and new. You don't have to prioritize (i.e., begin with your "best" friend).

  - Put an "F" next to any person who is a family member.

  - Put an "O" (for old friend) next to any person who has been your friend for five years or more.

  - Put an "N" next to any person who is a new friend (has been your friend for five years or less).

  - Think of some decisions you make. How much input does each one of these people have in your decision-making process? Give each person on your list a percentage of stock in your decision-making process. Also, give yourself some of the stock. Your total must equal one hundred percent for each decision.

  - Did you list anyone because you thought you *had* to? If so, cross that person off your list.

  - Is anyone on your list a crazymaker? If so, list some ways this person has affected your life in negative (and positive) ways.

- If we have been entangled with a crazymaker for a long time, getting detached may take some work. Disengaging may require rehearsal. One way of doing this is by writing an imaginary dialogue with your crazymaker. Written dialogues can be used as a form of interior role-playing, in which we say no to a crazymaker and try to establish some boundaries with her or him. Written dialogues are also time-honored ways of putting ourselves inside the shoes of someone with whom we are in conflict or of someone whom we love.

Process: Sit quietly, relax. Do some deep breathing. Write the name of a crazymaker with whom you need to dialogue. Then just reflect on the person: what they look like and how you feel with him or her. Next, after a period of quiet, write a dialogue with the person. Write a question that you want to ask them or a statement you need to make to the person. Then write the person's response. Sometimes a good place to begin with a crazymaker is with a statement of the boundary you want to establish. Let it flow where it will. Keep writing until you have completed the conversation. Then ask yourself if you need to take any action in regard to this relationship.

- If you work with someone with whom you frequently become frustrated, tell yourself that person is doing the best she or he can do. If we change what we think, we'll change our feelings. Remember that just because you must work with a crazymaker, you do not have to bring them home with you. Leave the frustrations this person causes you at the job site.

- Spend time with the people you care about. We often get so busy that we don't give ourselves the joy of being with the people we love.

To know what you prefer
instead of humbly saying
"Amen"
To what the world tells you
you ought to prefer,
Is to have kept your soul alive.

Robert Louis Stevenson

Reconciliation

I have an old friend whom I first met when we were in kindergarten. Over the years, our friendship grew, and she became a powerful influence in my life. In fact, this person gradually became like a member of my family. She spent holidays at my family's home and vacationed with us nearly every summer.

Over thirty-eight years, our friendship flourished. Then, suddenly it seemed, she shut me out. We became almost strangers. She no longer had time for me, and when I would call her on the phone, her response felt hurried and curt. She did not want to vacation, go out to dinner, or do any of the activities that had become part of our routine.

I found myself helpless and lost. How would I find out what was wrong when she wouldn't even return my calls? All attempts to get answers failed. She shut herself off from me and aligned herself with another friend. There was no room for me.

Losing my friend felt like what I imagined divorce was like. In this crisis, I had a hard time seeing any light at the end of the tunnel. Thoughts and anxieties about the break constantly buzzed around in my head. Letting go of the pain seemed impossible. She had become a crazymaker in my head.

The healing took time. I couldn't change the hand that life dealt me in this situation, but I could determine the way I would play these cards. The old adage that pain makes us grow stronger took on meaning for me. I kept reminding myself that nothing comes without cost. "For the benefit of the flowers," the Jewish saying teaches, "we water the thorns, too." For much of this time of trauma, I was only aware of the thorns and the suffering. The grace of the moment eluded me. I found myself looking backward to see what had been or forward to see what could be.

I had other friends. They helped, but I still had to carry the pain and suffering. We each must own our unique pain. Then, hopefully, we can grow through it and be free of it. Katharine Hepburn once remarked, "As one goes through life, one learns that if you don't paddle your own canoe, you don't move." The price of this paddling was not slight. It required believing in myself and owning my own gifts and strengths. It called for a stretching to learn a new part of who I was and an awareness of gifts of which I had never been aware. As the old saying reminded me, "If you bring forth what is within you, what you bring forth will save you."

This friend of mine didn't speak to me for fifteen years. What I learned during all those years was that time has a way of easing the pain. I had to let go and open myself to new relationships. I had healed pretty well over this incident.

I had frequently pondered the stress principle, "Don't waste your time trying to befriend a mad dog." If someone chooses not to be in my life or does not want to respond in a way I would like, it is better to turn away and find healthier and more positive people. Even though I still cared for my friend, I realized that caring for her didn't mean being miserable over her, and it didn't mean that I had to be in pain forever. An old Russian proverb reminds us, "When you live next to the cemetery, you can't cry for everyone who dies."

This story has an ending. I had invited some people over for dinner and went to the market to purchase the food for the meal. Grocery stores are always an experience for me. I always seem to get into the wrong line—

the one where someone needs a price check or a person didn't bring enough money and so has to decide which items she or he doesn't really want.

On this occasion the cashier announced that the person in front of me was the last one she would serve. I gave my usual response, thanking her, and then pushed my cart to another aisle. Not really looking at where I was going, I rammed my cart into another person's. I looked and saw that it was my old friend.

I smiled. "Hi. How are you?"

"Good. How are you?"

Shocked, I looked around and said, "Are you talking to me?" This began a twenty-minute conversation.

I will always be grateful for those twenty minutes. Many healing words were spoken. I asked her why she spoke this time. After all, for fifteen years, she had never responded when I called her on the phone or greeted her in person.

She told me that when I looked at her I smiled.

As I drove home from the store, I could not help but smile again and wonder at the power of eye contact and a smile! Smiles are blessings we give to each other. They are ways we send positive blessings to another's heart and console each other. And they help the one who smiles too!

The story about the old friend is still being written. We have had lunch together a few times since this meeting. Healing has begun. No, it's not the old friendship. Having been hurt once, I am proceeding slowly and cautiously. But at least we can speak. And we have shared some moments of laughter. We are creating some new memories. Phyllis Diller was certainly right when she said, "A smile is a curve that sets everything straight."

A SAD SOUL CAN KILL YOU QUICKER,

FAR QUICKER, THAN A GERM.

John Steinbeck

So Long, Mary

Throughout my life, I have spent a lot of time trying to figure out how to maintain my cool while the world swirls around me, especially when I'm with people who seem to affect me with their moods—both good and bad. I was raised with the idea that I should get along with everyone and, if I didn't like someone (or even if I liked them but they drove me nuts), I should still be able to be gracious and calm around them.

Over the years, I've come across lots of people who tax my inner reserves. Folks who talk incessantly or who seem to be in constant motion can be quite a challenge for this quiet introvert. It also takes as much energy for me to be around people who are negative or gossiping, as well as those who demand constant attention.

Years ago I had a new friend who seemed to be perfect for me. Mary had moved from the Washington, D.C., area about a year before we met. She was intelligent, well read, and interested in many of the things that interested me. We did a lot together. We went on retreats, discussed books, and commiserated with each other about ending up in a small town after both of us had lived in major metropolitan areas. She introduced me to new spiritual writers and storytellers. I was glad to have a friend like Mary who, I thought, shared so many of my values and interests. However, after awhile, I began feeling uncomfortable about the relationship. Nothing I could put my finger on, except my husband would periodically comment that if Mary stressed me so, why did I stay friends.

Mary was a teacher by training who now worked as a clerk for a small consulting firm. They specialized in human resource management and were very successful. She had moved from a metropolitan area to our small town two years before and was not able to find a teaching position, so ended up taking this clerical position. Over the months, she began to complain more and more about the other employees in her office. She had a particular dislike for one of the owners. She seemed obsessed with this person's perceived shortcomings.

When we were together, no matter what we were doing, Mary would always have a comment or two about her boss. Her remarks would be bitter, sarcastic, and sometimes even vicious. Many times she would call me at odd hours. Some mornings the phone would ring at 6:00 a.m.

"I know you and your husband get up early, so I thought it okay to call. I have to tell you what happened last night with my boss. She is so dysfunctional. I just don't know what to do." Then she would begin a vitriolic recitation of her boss's stupidity.

Any suggestions I tried to offer would be lost in her ranting. She, of course, would never sense from the icy tone of my voice that a 6:00 a.m. phone call was unacceptable. But I never said anything because, as a friend, I thought I should be available to her any time. However, the now increased phone calls were creating some stress between my husband and me.

Finally, one day all that false loyalty that I thought I owed Mary as a friend—maybe even blind devotion—abruptly vanished. I had had enough. During a time in which I was going through a painful experience, we met for lunch along with a mutual friend, Kathy. It was my birthday, and I was looking forward to being with supportive friends. We met at a popular restaurant that had great bagels, muffins, and other comfort food. Kathy was very much an earth mother, so I looked forward to an hour or so of a sympathetic ear and lots of support. It didn't happen.

Without asking us, Mary invited another woman who was eating alone at the restaurant to join us for lunch. Mary knew this woman, but Kathy and I did not. The newcomer seemed nice, and generally I wouldn't have minded. But it was my birthday lunch, and I needed to be alone with Mary and Kathy. Then, sure enough, during the entire meal, Mary went on and on about how dysfunctional the firm's owners were. At one point I asked her why she stayed.

"You just don't understand. I have to because I need the job," she snapped.

Hurt and frustrated, I sat quietly through the rest of my birthday lunch. I realized I didn't want to be there. My shoulders had tightened and my neck had grown stiff. I didn't want to listen to Mary's complaints anymore. Instead of a happy respite from the painful mess in my life, I felt snared again in Mary's endless, obsessive anger. Enough was enough.

After I left, I thought about what Mary and I each contributed to our relationship, and what we received from being with each other. At last, I decided that being with Mary was not what I wanted in a friendship, and that I didn't need to stay out of any sense of loyalty.

At the time, the decision to not see her anymore was difficult because I was still worried about her thinking badly of me. I was also saddened over ending a friendship that I thought had so much potential. However, the stress the relationship caused me far outweighed concerns about her opinion of me. I could choose the relationships that were supportive and nurturing. I did not need to stay in those that weren't. Enough craziness invaded my life uninvited; I didn't need to put down the welcome mat to the stress Mary always dragged in.

Since then, I've been fairly alert to those folks who drain my energy reserves. I now try to listen to my inner voice of caution when it tells me something just doesn't feel right about a particular person. Also, I have learned that relationships don't have to be all or nothing. Friends don't have to be joined at the hip or nonexistent. I am cautious when I notice people not respecting my time or if the relationship lacks mutuality. And when someone is continually in a crisis, after initial attempts at helping, I tend to disengage.

Sometimes my friends can drag me down a bit, and I'm sure I can do the same to them. A couple of my friends are extroverts who tend to chatter when they're nervous or when a lot is going on in their lives. I have learned to stay grounded when I'm with them and let them know when I need a break. I can still get caught in the whirlwind, but usually I can pull myself out and get my feet on the ground again.

It took me a while to recognize crazymakers in my life. I had always thought that I was the one who couldn't cope. My experience with Mary helped me understand that there are certain people I just don't need to be around.

Rosalie Hooper-Thomas

YOU ARE LOOKING AT THE FACE OF THE PERSON WHO IS RESPONSIBLE FOR YOUR HAPPINESS TODAY.

John Powell

WAY 6 :

Reach Out to Kindred Spirits

EVERY BLADE OF GRASS HAS ITS
ANGEL THAT BENDS OVER IT AND
WHISPERS, "GROW, GROW."

The Talmud

Social ties are so vital that some researchers link good health to having a circle of supportive friends and family. Positive relationships can reduce stress. Having someone to turn to and share our stories with can have a profound effect upon our mental and physical health. We all need people in our lives who are healthy, positive, and nurturing for us. People who like us. People who care about us. As the Gaelic proverb says, "It's in the shadow of each other that the people live." To keep our balance, we all need relationships with family, friends, and significant people.

Having a pet is also a good stress-reducer. Companion animals offer us unconditional acceptance. Indeed, studies have shown that people who own pets tend to live longer. Participating in social groups— community organizations, churches, card clubs, softball teams—can reduce stress too.

If one does not have a helpful support system, going to a mental health counselor is often money well spent. A whole body of research tells us that counseling—even apart from exercise or modification of diet—can reduce the risk of heart attacks. Other research suggests that staying connected in healthy relationships may protect against depression and increase the odds of surviving a heart attack. Participating in healthy relationships can even decrease the risk of catching a cold. In short, companionship is good medicine, whereas isolating ourselves from life-giving people can increase our stress to toxic levels.

A psychologist at the University of Michigan, Barbara Fredrickson, has studied happiness extensively. Not surprisingly, she has discovered that happiness is a good thing! Fredrickson showed how happiness is an antidote to stress. Her studies also point out how happiness can lower pulse rates and can alleviate anxiety, which can cause cardiovascular damage. She theorizes that positive emotions broaden the mind's ability to think. When we hold on to negative emotions we narrow our thoughts because they are essentially a response to some perceived threat on which our mind is concentrating. Happiness allows the mind to wander, invent, and be creative. Happy and healthy is a smart way to live.

Friends make us happy, and happiness is a great way to make friends. We all like to be around happy, positive people. Fredrickson maintains, "Happy people draw others to them." She also states, "Happiness begets happiness because other people find you reasonable and exciting, and that helps you continue to feel good."

So, reach out to kindred spirits!

FAITHFUL FRIENDS ARE A STURDY

SHELTER:

WHOEVER FINDS ONE HAS FOUND A

TREASURE.

FAITHFUL FRIENDS ARE LIFE-SAVING

MEDICINE.

Ecclesiasticus

Reach Out to Kindred Spirits

- Make time for people you care about. When was the last time you had a long visit with your best friend?
  - Call a person you know would love to hear from you.
  - Jot a note to a lonely person or to someone who lives alone.
- Hug five people you love. Even if they try to push you away (teenagers often do this), hug them anyway. They will carry the hug in their heart.
- Give someone a bouquet of fresh flowers or some homegrown vegetables from your garden. The gift will come back a hundredfold.
- Join a book club or sign up for a class at a nearby college. It will be a way to connect and meet other people.

- Start a conversation with someone you don't know at your church, at the grocery store, or in an airport. Greet a stranger with a compliment. That's how we learn to reach out to others.

- Invite to your home for dinner a person to whom you don't owe anything.

FRIENDSHIP IS A MIRACLE BY WHICH
A PERSON CONSENTS TO VIEW FROM
A CERTAIN DISTANCE, AND WITHOUT
COMING ANY NEARER, THE VERY
BEING WHO IS NECESSARY TO HIM AS
FOOD.

Simone Weil

Helena's Mom

Recently I had the privilege of counseling Helena, a lovely, intelligent, and happy ten-year-old child. She was an only child of loving parents. In any case, the principal of the school she attended called me and asked that I see her.

Recently, her grandparents, whom she was very close to, had both died within two days of each other. Helena's aunt died a month later of complications from a kidney transplant operation. Helena's mother, Joanna, was on the list for a heart transplant, double lung transplant, and a kidney transplant. The principal wondered, how much could a ten-year-old child take?

Helena only knew that her mother as sick. She had become accustomed to her mother going to hospitals in Boston, Pittsburgh, and Albany and did not think of this as unusual. Her mother was on a medication that allowed only a six-minute time frame when it needed to be replaced. Helena knew how to change the medication and did it with the ease of an adult nurse. Joanna would accompany Helena to the counseling sessions in a wheelchair. The wheelchair, too, was second nature to the family.

One Thursday I received a phone call from Helena, telling me that her mother had been taken to the hospital. I thought the phone call was unusual since Joanna was taken to the hospital frequently. I asked Helena what she wanted me to do. She said, "I just needed to hear your voice."

Later that evening I went to the hospital to see what was going on. I was directed to the waiting area on the third floor. Helena spotted me and ran over and hugged me. This was the delightful ten-year-old I knew.

Helena asked me to come with her to her mother's room. As we drew near the bed, Helena took her mother's hand. She told her mother that I was there. I assured Joanna that we were praying for her and were all taking care of each other. Most especially, we were caring for her daughter. Joanna nodded as I spoke to her.

After several hours I decided to leave the hospital. The number of family members was swelling, and the support they were giving each other was evident. Helena did not understand why I was leaving. I gave her my home phone number and told her to feel free to call me in the middle of the night if she needed to. I also said I would be back in the morning.

The next morning I checked with my secretary and was told that all life supports would be removed from Joanna about 11:30 a.m. Helena had left a message asking me to be present.

As I got off the elevator, Helena ran over to me and started to cry. "My mother is going to die. My mother is going to die today."

The family seemed confused as to why Helena had not understood the seriousness of her mother's condition. But Helena was only ten years old and had grown accustomed to her mom being in the hospital and then always returning home.

The next few hours were difficult for the family members as they all went in and said their good-byes. A beautiful prayer service and a ritual of having family members bless Joanna helped all of us prepare to let her go.

Joanna died peacefully around 12:20 in the afternoon with her daughter, husband, and extended family surrounding her. Sadness, stress, and grief would live with this family for a good while, but they had reserves of love that would help them heal. And I promised Helena that I would be there for her whenever she needed me.

No matter what accomplishments you achieve, somebody helped you.

Althea Gibson

A Friend Indeed

I am a recovering alcoholic. I can say those words easily these days—easily, not publicly—but years ago, at the beginning, I choked on those words. A compassionate counselor gently guided me to admit that I, indeed, did have a drinking problem. However, the early days were hard, very hard. I might have admitted that I had a problem, but it took me a while to accept it. I went through outpatient treatment and during that time began going to meetings of Alcoholics Anonymous.

My first meeting was on a Sunday at a downtown recovery club. I went because my counselors in treatment told me to. I still felt that I didn't belong because the meeting was filled with people whose lives were really unmanageable. People who had lost their jobs, lost their marriages, and some who had lost their freedom with several DWIs. Many people attended because they were sent there by the courts. There were poor, low class people there—at least that is what they seemed in my eyes.

You see, I was a professional from a wealthy, white suburb. I was still married, still working, and had never been stopped by the police for drinking and driving. Of course, that's not to say my marriage was any good or that I was doing well at work, or hadn't driven while drinking. But all was manageable. All was in good order. Or so I thought.

Anyway, at the Sunday meeting, I occasionally would speak up, usually about how miserable I was. Nobody there could really understand all the problems I had. Nobody could understand how much pain I was in. *I* had special problems. *I* had a particularly difficult childhood. *I* was under such stress. However, I was still able to maintain in spite of it all. Anyway, nobody could really understand.

As the weeks passed by, I started to crawl out of my self-absorption and noticed a slim, somewhat smallish African-American man who was always at the meeting. His clothes were old and his pants were held up with a rope for a belt. He wore a frayed gray sport coat and always a dark gray fedora. After he sat down, he would take the hat off and gently, precisely set it down on the table at his place. I noticed that he generally wouldn't say much. He did tell us he was sent to AA by the courts. I noticed him, but I knew I didn't have anything in common with him. I could feel sorry for him and his circumstances, but no way did I think we had anything in common.

After a while, this gentle, frail man began to talk. He spoke of being lonely and afraid, of never feeling as if he belonged anywhere. For him, the pain of his loneliness and fear was so bad that the only thing that helped him forget, for just a moment, was a drink. And not just one drink. He knew that after the drinking he felt worse, but he just couldn't help himself. I was stunned! This inner city black man with a rope for a belt spoke of my same loneliness, my same fear, and my same pain. How did he know? And so I began listening more closely to him and to the others. I had found folks who not only were feeling what I was feeling, but who readily admitted and accepted their alcoholism.

As the weeks went on in those early days, I added a couple of AA meetings closer to home. I stopped going to the Sunday meeting downtown. A women's meeting was especially helpful to me because we could talk about issues that might not have been appropriate at a general meeting. And these women were astute at keeping me honest. At this meeting, I found the woman who was to become my sponsor. She was tough on me. Sometimes even making me mad. But she knew what alcoholism was all about, and she knew what was needed for me to stay on the path of recovery.

Five years later, I moved away from the city where I got sober. I found new meetings and a new sponsor. I continued to go to meetings weekly to be with folks who understood not how miserable my life was, but who knew what was needed to stay sober. When my days got too stressed from work, a meeting refocused me on the things I needed to do to keep some balance in my life. When I got out of sorts, not knowing what was wrong, something that someone said at a meeting brought insight and clarity and peace.

A friend once questioned my need to go to meetings after all these years. "Surely," he said, "you won't drink again, will you? Why do you still go to meetings?" I assured him that I had no intention of drinking, but being with folks who knew the insidious nature of alcoholism and the stresses of alcoholics helped keep me on track and guided me on my path of serenity, the ultimate goal of recovery.

My recovery group is not the only group that supplies support and insight for daily living. Many of my friends provide the same role. I know that when I do get caught up in the stress of living or when I seem to come up against a crisis, I am now open to reaching out to those who will hear me and hold me with their love and support. And I owe at least some of the credit to a gentle, slim black man who broke through my isolating

haze with his own cry of pain. Bless him. We may find
kindred spirits where we least expect.

Delores T.

A FRIEND IS SOMEONE WHO WALKS
IN WHEN THE REST OF THE WORLD
WALKS OUT.

Walter Winchell

Care for Your Body and Your Body Will Care for You

SOLVITUR AMBULANDO . . . . IT IS
SOLVED BY WALKING.

Augustine of Hippo

Most of us know that we carry much of our stress in our bodies. When we are stressed our blood pressure rises, our shoulders stiffen, our stomach ties in knots, and our breathing quickens. Our immune system becomes suppressed, so we tend to become ill more easily. Stress has been known to hasten diabetes and certainly heart trouble too.

Not so surprisingly, our bodies need not be victims of stress. Rather, our bodies can actually help us cope with all the tension and worry. Three practices have been shown to be particularly effective in dealing with stress: deep breathing, exercise, and rest. Each practice is readily available, far less expensive than medicines and doctor visits, and natural to everyone.

Remember when you were a kid, crying because you got pitched off of your bicycle? Sobs wracked your little body as you cried for mom or dad to stop the bleeding and the hurting of your scraped knees and elbows. You could barely breathe between the sobs. Invariably, we were told to take some deep breaths. As our parent held us our sobs would subside to whimpers, and our breathing would slowly come closer to normal. Unfortunately, as we have grown up, most of us start breathing like that hurt child we once were—except when we are sleeping. Only in the land of nod do we inhale all the way down to the bottom of our diaphragm.

Breathing deeply is the first simple technique for reducing stress. Many of us need to relearn deep breathing. Most of us have forgotten how to breathe. As a matter of course, we tend to take short shallow breaths, and our body responds with an increase in heart rate, blood pressure, and fear hormones. The mind responds with negativity and fantasies of loneliness and unworthiness.

Deep breathing is essential for health and easing stress. In many respects, it is the single most effective way to combat stress. Deep breathing relaxes us when we are panicked or feel fear. It distracts us from pain and anxiety and gives us an energy boost. It also sharpens our awareness. Deep breathing slows us down to appreciate the moment in front of us.

We inhale and exhale more than ten million times a year. At a resting pace, we breathe in and out about twenty times every minute. So we have plenty of time to practice breathing. When the breath is long and slow, the body becomes peaceful and relaxed. The mind can rest.

Engaging in activity is the second way our body can help us deal with stress. Notice, the emphasis here is on activity, not necessarily vigorous exercise or participation in sports. Research has shown that even twenty minutes a day of activity can ease our mind and help our body at the same time. Activities such as taking the stairs instead of the elevator, walking to the office from the end of the parking lot, working in a garden, strolling with our dog around the block, and cleaning the attic can all burn calories, jump start our endorphins (the body's natural painkillers), tone our muscles, increase our circulation, and help us sleep better.

While games like golf, tennis, and racquetball are great exercise, trying to find time, line up people to play with, and reserve a course or court may actually increase our stress. Then too, if we are highly competitive, playing can put even more pressure on us. If you can work in an exercise program, fine, otherwise seek small ways of being active.

One last word on activity and stress reduction. When you are walking, just walk and be aware of your surroundings. When you clean, clean. When you garden, just be in the garden. During times of activity, learn to just engage in the activity—not use the time to plan or worry. The activity time should be just that: time for activity. Give yourself a break, and chances are that when you do return to work you will come back refreshed and ready.

The final simple stress reducing technique is so basic: Get enough rest. Without sufficient rest, stress finds us an easy target. Restful sleep does not only refresh the body but is essential for our mental health. Mark Mahoward, director of Minnesota Regional Sleep Disorders Center, stated, "We were raised to believe that sleep deprivation is a badge of honor. People never brag about how much sleep they've gotten, but they brag about how little sleep they've gotten."

The National Sleep Foundation research indicates that sleep needs vary by age and from person to person, but offers some general guidelines:

Toddlers: 11 hours plus a two-hour nap during the day.

Preschoolers: 11 to 12 hours. Half of preschoolers also nap during the day.

School-aged children: About 10 hours.

Teens: Average of 9 hours. Studies show that most get far less than that.

Adults: Generally eight hours or more. Needs vary. The average adult sleeps six hours and fifty-four minutes on weeknights and seven hours, thirty-four minutes on weekends.

We know that when people get enough sleep they feel mental clarity, whereas people become more confused and emotional when they are sleep deprived. If we are deprived of sleep and something strikes us as funny, we may get silly and giggly. If something strikes us as sad, we are more likely to cry. It is harder to channel feelings of frustration and anger if we have not had enough sleep. Students who are tired are more likely to doze off in class and are less able to concentrate, learn, and solve problems. People who fall asleep while driving cars cause accidents and deaths.

So having a sleep plan and being faithful to it are important. Going to bed at the same time each night is a helpful thing. It is better not to drink caffeine or to exercise or play computer games before going to bed. These cause us to perk up. Keeping our bodies on schedule is important. Limiting the exposure to light in the late evening and increasing it in the morning helps the body clock stay on track.

These three ways of caring for our body require some discipline, but they are less expensive than anti-hypertensive drugs and antidepressants, can be done with household equipment, and are simple enough for anyone. Best of all, they are wonderfully effective tools to cope with stress.

BRINGING AWARENESS TO OUR BREATHING, WE REMIND OURSELVES THAT WE ARE HERE NOW, SO WE MIGHT AS WELL BE FULLY AWAKE FOR WHATEVER IS ALREADY HAPPENING.

Jon Kabat-Zinn

Care for Your Body and Your Body Will Care for You

- We can learn this technique. Breathing plays an essential role in calming and focusing the mind and body. Breathe as deeply as you can comfortably do so. Invite your breath to fill the lower parts of your lungs, pushing out the diaphragm, thus lifting your stomach. Breathe slowly and deeply.

  As you breathe out, count "1."

  As you breathe in, say "and."

  As you breathe out, count "2."

As you breathe in, say "and."

Continue through 4, then return again to 1.

If you become distracted or lose count, gently return to 1 and begin again. Eventually, just stop the counting and focus on your deep breathing; if you become distracted, pick up the breathing once again. This little exercise can be repeated throughout a day: waiting for a traffic light to change; waiting to pick your child up at school; waiting to check out groceries. Take a few breaths before beginning your dinner and savor what you are about to eat.

- Find twenty minutes each day for activity. Here is one way to set aside the time. First, divide a piece of paper into seven columns. In each column, write down a rough schedule for each day—not an ideal one, but what you usually do. When you have roughed out the schedule, note any activity that you are already doing: for example, walking from your car to the office or taking a coffee break in the morning. Finally, see how you can turn up the level of activity, so that day by day you get a bit more exercise. For example, instead of finding a parking place as close to the door as possible, park at the other end of the lot. Instead of going for coffee, take a fifteen-minute walk outside or up and down some indoor stairs. Instead of sending as many e-mails, walk to people's offices more often. Every morning go for a brief walk and then as you feel better, take a faster walk. In other words, increase your activity.

- Every day give yourself a three-minute relaxation break. Take in a deep breath and hold it. While you are holding your breath, tense up a group of muscles, such as the muscles in your face, arms, or legs. As you breathe out, relax the tensed muscles and feel the tension slip away.

- Get a good night's sleep.
  - Take a warm bath or listen to soothing music.
  - Keep a regular routine. Go to bed and wake up at the same time every day whether you are tired or not.
  - Save your bed for sleep. Don't eat or watch TV in bed.
  - If you can't sleep, get up, go into another room, and read, write in your journal, or do a crossword puzzle.
- If you already have an exercise program, but your stress level is still too high, ask yourself these questions: Is exercise stressing me out? Has it become work? Do I see it as just another thing I have to do or as a time to feel good about my body and to ease my mind? Am I so competitive that I experience exercise as just another test of myself? If your answer is yes to any of these questions, consider (a) altering your exercise plan to something less competitive or driven and/or (b) concentrating on just enjoying the activity for itself.

AFOOT AND LIGHT-HEARTED I TAKE

TO THE OPEN ROAD,

HEALTHY, FREE, THE WORLD

BEFORE ME.

Walt Whitman

Taking a Walk

Along with thousands of other walkers, my friend Ellen, my wife Joyce, and I did some light warm-up aerobics in preparation for the annual AIDS Walk Wisconsin. I was glad that Ellen was joining Joyce and me for the walk not only because the AIDS Resource Center was a good cause, but more so because going on the walk signaled a radical shift in Ellen's life. When I asked her about sponsoring me, she had declared her intention of walking with us. Hearing the surprise in my voice, she told me about the changes in her life since the last time we had talked.

"When I walked into Frank's office, I knew that I was history. We had been wrangling over every design that I sent him. The straw that broke this camel's back was when he tried to demote me because I wouldn't do a sexy cover for an ad brochure. It was sexist and trashy. I just wouldn't do it like that. It would be bad for our image, the company we designed for, and for me personally. I didn't want to be associated with that kind of junk. Anyway, he handed me a letter that said I was fired or I could resign. The severance was bigger if I resigned. He told me that I had to decide then and there. So I signed the resignation. He gave me two hours to leave the building. That, after almost ten years with the company.

"I waited until I got outside to cry. It was a mixture of anger, bitterness, hurt, and embarrassment. With twenty-twenty hindsight, I think I was secretly relieved too. My design projects accounted for almost a quarter of the company's income, but I was too big a threat to Frank. Like so many managers in the company, he had long ago risen to the level of his incompetence. Working for such a nincompoop had been a pain for nearly a year. I had to take blood pressure medicine. I'd gained thirty-three pounds and hadn't slept well in weeks. Physically I was a wreck and getting worse.

"If finances hadn't been so tight, I would have been more relieved. The job market in Milwaukee for graphic designers wasn't great at all. Most of the companies wanted cheap newcomers. With Kevin still in college, we needed my income, so I started looking. We would be okay for a while, but not indefinitely.

"And, I had just turned the big five-zero, 50. The first couple of interviews I managed to line up were with people half my age. They clearly seemed intimidated. I got the feeling that finding a full-time position with a firm was going to take longer than I guessed. The whole mess was really getting to me. I found myself eating too much and, after a routine visit to my doctor, I knew that my blood pressure was reaching a dangerous level.

"So, I made two decisions. First, I decided to freelance, at least until I could find a full-time job. The second decision has proven to be even more important in the long run. I decided to join Weight Watchers. I figured that if it were good enough for my friend Alice, who lost nearly eighty pounds, it would sure be good for me. Otherwise I might be dead or have a stroke sooner rather than later.

"Thankfully Ted, agreed and was supportive. I think he was relieved too. All the stress made me grumpy and distracted, besides making me physically unhealthy. I started counting my points, cooking differently. Actually, at the start, a lot of my frustrated creative energy got put into trying new, low-cal recipes. Some were great and others awful. Ted was so tolerant, good husband that he is.

"Weight Watchers tells you to be active at least twenty minutes a day. Freelancing made that easy. After working on a project for an hour, I'd get up and vacuum the living room. I got on a regular cleaning schedule. My house hasn't been that clean in years. And I started walking every day. The first week I thought I would die. Twenty minutes seemed like an eternity. I bet I walked only about half a mile. You know though, when I got home, my legs hurt, but I felt better.

"Pretty soon I was walking for thirty minutes, then an hour when I could. And I always felt better. The pounds came off—more slowly than I would have liked—but I lost all the same. But you know the best part? I started having more energy, I slept better, and I stopped worrying so much. As a result, I think I'm doing the best design work I've done in years.

"When I hit my goal weight, I walked into the doctor's office knowing that I could get off my blood pressure medicine. She was shocked out of her mind. First time I ever saw her speechless. Sure enough, my pressure was great. No more money for meds. I feel great.

"I still don't have a full-time job, but freelancing is keeping us afloat. If I get stuck on a project or start stewing over something, I get out the vacuum and clean house or better yet lace up my sneakers and head out for a walk."

A month after our conversation, here we stood at the starting line for the AIDS Walk. Ellen looked great in body and in spirit. As soon as the honorary chair blew the whistle, we all started walking. The sun showed brightly. A cool breeze wafted off Lake Michigan. But the best feeling of all came from the wonderful transformation in our friend, Ellen.

Carl Koch

I HAVE TWO DOCTORS—MY LEFT

LEG AND MY RIGHT.

Anonymous

Home

During a retreat, Rose—not her real name—told this story about keeping life in balance through rest, exercise, and readjusting priorities.

When Dave walked into the house, I knew that something terrible had happened. Dave dragged in his bags and dropped them on the floor in the hallway. His face was ashen. His eyes just stared.

First I gave Dave a quick kiss and a tight hug, then I asked him, "Dave, what happened? You look like hell."

Dave didn't even attempt a weak smile. He shook his head as if trying to clear his head.

I told him to go take a shower and clean up. Then we could eat something. Caitlin, our daughter, was at play practice, and A.J., our son, had already eaten.

I watched Dave slowly climb the stairs. As I warmed up the lasagna and made Dave's salad, worry and fear hit. What could have happened?

Dave took a long shower. When he sat down, he looked a little bit better.

I filled him in on what had happened with the kids and at my work, waiting until he had eaten before I asked again, "Okay, Dave, what happened?"

"I drove all the way through Chicago and didn't realize it until I was in Gary. The only reason I knew that I'd hit Gary was I hit the warning strip on the side of the expressway. If it hadn't woke me up, I would have gone off the road."

"My God, Dave. Haven't you been sleeping again?"

"I'm just so tired, Rose. The better business is going, the more pressure I'm under. And I just get more and more tired. I can't go on this way."

I knew that he couldn't keep up the pace. Dave was forty-one, but looked ten years older. I urged him to go to bed, and then told him, "You're taking tomorrow off."

"I can't. I have a meeting with a new account at 11:00, and . . . ."

"No, Dave," I cut him off. "You're not. The world won't stop if you finally take care of yourself for once. I'll take the day off too. I want you around for Sarah's performance a month from now, A.J.'s graduation, and us as old folks together."

"Okay" was all Dave said in reply. Now I knew that Dave had hit a wall. Before tonight, Dave would never admit that he could take time off.

The irony of the situation was inescapable. Three years ago Dave had left the high-pressure corporation he had worked at. As a rising star in the company, Dave had been expected to work up to one hundred hours per week. For a few years, Dave and I put up with this. The pay and perks were great. Then during Dave's last year, he started leaving work later and later. He spent most Saturdays answering e-mails and working at his laptop. I hit the ceiling when Dave insisted that he bring his pager, cell phone, and laptop on vacation. I was fed up with Dave, the company, and the fact that I felt like a single parent.

In fact, Dave had been thinking about a move too. He decided to set up his own consulting firm, work more from home, and take only the jobs he wanted. And for the first eighteen months all had gone smoothly. Gradually though, Dave's competence and hard work had become his enemies. His services were in growing demand. As an independent engineering consultant, he feared turning jobs down because he didn't know what work might come his way next. So he took on more projects than he could handle. Soon, Dave worked as hard and long as he had at his old company. He slept badly and never long enough, always thinking about the next project and all he had to get done. He seldom jogged anymore, abandoning the one form of exercise that he had begun after leaving the company.

When I challenged him about the stress he was under and his return to the same grind, he would straighten up, make some glib remark about being Superman, and quickly change the subject. After what he said about not remembering the drive through Chicago, I realized that Dave was, once again, at the breaking point.

To my surprise, Dave slept soundly that night. I noticed that he had turned off his pager, his cell phone, and had left the laptop in the hall downstairs. When I slipped out of bed in the morning, Dave simply rolled over.

Right at 8:00, I called our family doctor and close friend, Bill, and begged for an appointment that day for Dave. Bill had his receptionist fit Dave in.

It took some firm reasoning on my part, but I managed to get Dave to Bill's office at 2:00. I felt a little foolish driving my husband to the doctor's office, but I was too worried not to.

Dave told me later that day what Bill said after his exam. "You're too young to have the kind of blood pressure you've got. I don't know what you're doing to yourself, but it isn't good. Now, you've got three choices, Dave. You can get out of the meat grinder you're in. Two, you can change the situation. Or, three, you can change your attitude and the way you're dealing with things.

"I don't know which of the three will work best. You need to do something. I can give you something to help you sleep, but I'd rather not. But if you don't get better sleep, you'll either be in here again soon or end up on a guardrail somewhere. And, you better start getting some exercise. It's up to you, but I'm glad Rose dragged you in today."

As we drove home, I waited for Dave to tell me what Bill said. When I couldn't stand it, I asked, "Well?"

"Well what?"

"What did Bill say?" He could be so maddening sometimes.

"He told me to tell you to drive to school to pick up the kids, to pick up some subs and soda, and then for us to go to the river for a picnic."

I liked what I heard, but didn't feel like joking. "Yeah, right. That's a good start though. But what else?"

"He told me that I better sleep more and get more exercise."

"That it?"

"That's a lot. It's like turning my whole world around. But, hey, it's a small price to pay for growing into elderhood with you. Pull over there. Stop."

He scared me half to death, but I pulled over. Dave undid his seatbelt, slid over, and kissed me like he did when we first got married.

"Wow," I told him, "I'm going to take you to the doctor more often."

"No you're not," Dave said. "This is it. I can get my life sane again. We might not have as much money, but I'll never drive through Chicago again and not remember it."

GOD RESTED ON THE SEVENTH DAY FROM ALL THE WORK OF CREATION. SO GOD BLESSED THE SEVENTH DAY AND MADE IT HOLY, BECAUSE ON THAT DAY GOD RESTED FROM ALL THE EFFORT OF CREATING THE WORLD.

Book of Genesis

WAY 8 :

Have Fun!

WE DON'T HAVE TO BE HAPPY TO
LAUGH. WE HAVE TO LAUGH TO BE
HAPPY.

William James

Once upon a time, a Zen story goes, a man was crossing a field and encountered a tiger. Running away, he came to a great cliff and caught hold of a root and swung over the edge of the cliff. But at the bottom of the cliff was another tiger.

Soon two little mice came along and began to gnaw on the vine. The man looked in terror at the tiger below. But then he saw a strawberry vine. He picked the strawberry and ate it. How delicious it was.

Once we begin to accept an inevitable situation, we can choose to transform it. When we recall these situations later they can even bring us laughter and joy. Think of the many gatherings—class reunions, anniversary celebrations, holidays—around which these situations are shared. Humor is a reaction to incongruity, to a discrepancy between what we expected and what we experience. The man still hung from the vine, tigers

99

waited above and below, but the strawberry was sweet. We take pleasure as we can. It doesn't solve all our problems, but it keeps the terror at bay.

Fun isn't reserved for children, clowns, and fools. Fun provides a stimulus that keeps people going. It is the connection we share with others. When people are having fun, they forget their troubles and concerns, and just enjoy the play. When people are having fun, they create more and begin to see other options. The perceptual world broadens, and people begin to listen differently and hear others. People who have fun live in the now and get all the energy from the moment at hand. It's hard to keep a stiff upper lip and smile at the same time.

When our lives get stressed and fun vanishes, our spirits suffer. The first gift to go is our sense of humor. We no longer laugh at our own absurdities or the craziness of others. We begin to search for dark, hidden meanings where there are no meanings at all. What an unhealthy state we are in! Robert Louis Stevenson said, "A happy man or woman is a radiant focus of good will, and their entrance into a room is as though another had been lighted." When we become too stressed and unable to laugh, all we bring is gloom.

Stress can actually be viewed as an invitation to risk being silly, to relax and enjoy the moment, and to remain in a healthy state. The word "silly" is originally from the Old English *saelig*, which meant "completely happy, joyful, and blessed." Silly was a blessing you wished upon those you loved.

What changed our thinking so that now we think of silly as being childish and immature? Sadly, we have come to accept that silly is for young children. No wonder our stress levels are out of whack.

We must find situations to put ourselves in which afford us the experiences of laughter, joy, and humor. We have to find ways to play or to even be like clowns, the professional fun-makers. Clowns work at having fun. They create opportunities for others to experience it. Clowns really are symbols of the child within all of us. We all want to play. "The human race has only one really effective weapon and that's laughter," Mark Twain wrote. "The moment it arises, all our hardnesses yield, all our irritations and resentments slip away, and a sunny spirit takes their place."

Laughing at ourselves is a sign that our spirit transcends the present trouble. We believe that this life is not all there is. We believe that our God will look after us. There is much evidence to suggest that people who can laugh in the face of adversity stand a better chance of recovery from disease than those who cannot laugh. Humor is a powerful sign for us that God does exist.

When we have a sense of humor, when we know how to play and have fun, we actually empower ourselves. Instead of making us less capable of dealing with reality, fun, humor, and play actually increase our efficiency and productivity. We can see new possibilities in difficult situations. We can gain some emotional distance from our problems and be in a better position to cope with them. We can change the perceptions of our circumstances before they change us. Phyllis Diller reminds us, "You've got to realize when all goes well, and everything is beautiful, you have no comedy. It's when somebody steps on the bride's train, or belches during the ceremony that you've got comedy!" And that comedy takes off the pressure, relieves the stress, and lets us laugh and enjoy.

LIFE WILL BRING YOU PAIN ALL BY
ITSELF. YOUR RESPONSIBILITY IS TO
CREATE JOY.

Milton Erickson

Have Fun!

- Give yourself a laughter break. Stop what you're doing and laugh out loud. Don't worry that someone will hear you. Laughter is contagious. Spread the joy.

- Start a treasure-trove of humorous stories, cartoons that you like, and jokes that cause you to roar. Take as your mission to share at least one goofy story or joke with one person every day. It will be good for you and for them.

- Look consciously for funny things that are happening right in front of you. Tune in to the moment and see the joy and laughter present. Remember, things are not as they are, but as we are. If we decide to see goodness and humor in life's situations, things will look that way.

- Send flowers to someone and don't sign your name.

- Write a letter to Santa Claus and thank him for last year's Christmas gifts.

- Proclaim today a "Play Day." Even if you have to work, play while you're there. Find ways to enjoy work.

+ Put cartoons on a bulletin board.

+ Share funny stories at coffee break time.

+ Begin staff meetings with an activity that helps everyone laugh.

+ Proclaim every Monday a "Smile Day." Anyone caught without a smile has to make a contribution to a worthy cause.

• Draw up a "Fun Contract" with yourself, which commits you to doing one fun thing every week—something pointless and playful. You might use some of the following Smollin's Prescription for Keeping Joy and Fun in Our Daily Life in your contract:

1. Believe you deserve to be happy.

2. Have fun daily.

3. Don't hang around negative people.

4. Be curious.

5. Live the present moment.

6. Smile, smile, and smile some more.

7. Expect the unexpected.

8. Be kind to others.

9. Every day give something away.

10. Laugh a lot each day—it's exercise.

11. Forgive—yourself and others.

12. Start each day anew.

13. Surround yourself with positive people.

14. Make some mistakes each day on purpose.

15. Laugh at yourself.

16. Keep a joy journal.

17. Take deep breathes during stressful events.

18. Learn something new each day.

19. Look for another way of doing something.

20. Count your blessings.

TAKE TIME TO WORK.

IT IS THE PRICE OF SUCCESS.

TAKE TIME TO THINK.

IT IS THE SOURCE OF POWER.

TAKE TIME TO LAUGH.

IT IS THE MUSIC OF THE SOUL.

Old English Prayer

A Big To-Do

The time for the annual Christmas cookie extravaganza had arrived once again. Mom and us kids traditionally spent an afternoon rolling out cookie dough, carefully picking which cookie cutter to use, and reminding each other not to eat the dough because it wasn't good for us. After the cookies had cooled, Mom frosted them and offered each one of us a batch to decorate any way we wanted. All the favorite decorations were laid out: colored balls, green sprinkles, and the favorite, longer brown sprinkles perfect for putting hair on the reindeer-shaped cookies.

Mom hummed along with the Christmas music as she watched the three of us decorate the cookies. She complimented each one of us on our designs. Once she had finished frosting the cookies, she sat back and began to enjoy watching the scene. Then a loud shrieking sound from my father in the other room shattered the peaceful moment.

"That's it! I've had enough!" he yelled. "I'm going to get every last one of them if it's the last thing I ever do!"

Mom looked at us. We knew exactly what Dad was yelling about. A gentle man by nature, my father had little tolerance for snakes or mice. Since it was the middle of a Wisconsin winter, we knew no snakes were slithering around the house. He must have found signs of mice. He hated mice.

"Honey, whatever is the matter?" Mom asked anyway.

"Mice. We've got a mouse in the laundry room. I found droppings by the dog dish. I've had it. Before you know it, we'll have families of mice living in our house. I'm going to take care of the little buggers once and for all."

Mom didn't like mice either, but felt that Dad got too excited about the whole situation. She tried her best to get Dad to settle down, but to no avail. Instead of coming to admire the creative cookies that us kids had made, Dad was too busy looking for the mousetraps and then setting them strategically in place.

We could tell that Dad's war on the mouse bothered Mom. What she really wanted was for him to relax and just enjoy the holiday activities with us. She thought that maybe if Dad could see just how ridiculous his behavior was he would not be quite so serious about his mission to eradicate all the mice in the universe.

As Mom looked around the table at the beautiful creations that we had made, a plan began to form. Last year a mouse had committed the ultimate insult, in my father's eyes. The wee and timorous beastie had left its droppings in the kids' toothbrush drawer. Mom was grossed out too, but Dad had gone ballistic.

Now Mom laughed as she whispered instructions to us. We all sneaked up to the master bedroom, bringing along the brown sprinkles. After glancing around to see if Dad was watching, she scattered several of the brown sprinkles in Dad's toothbrush drawer. We began to laugh as we imagined the coming events. The brown sprinkles looked just like mouse droppings. We all quickly left the area. Mom whispered that Beth should now implement Operation Mouse Revenge.

"Dad, come quick!" Beth screamed. "I think a mouse has been in your bathroom!"

Armed with an arsenal of mousetraps, Dad came running up the steps. He began ranting about how rotten mice were and how they must be wiped out of existence.

Mom now sprung her own trap. She ran into the master bathroom and asked what was wrong. We, of course, followed.

"I can't believe it!" my father bellowed. "The mice are even up here in our bathroom!"

"How can you be sure?" Mom asked innocently.

"Here's your evidence. The little guy left us a present in our toothbrush drawer!" He then pointed accusingly at the brown "droppings" in the drawer.

"What do you mean? How do you know those are mouse droppings?" Mom replied.

Dad rolled his eyes. "Anyone knows a mouse dropping when he sees it."

Mom winked at us kids and calmly walked over to the drawer. Glancing at Dad, she said, "I think you might be right. Maybe these are from a mouse. Let me check." With that, she quickly picked up several of the "droppings" and popped them into her mouth, making a big to-do about relishing the taste.

Dad's mouth dropped open, wondering if his wife had finally lost her mind. The three of us and Mom couldn't contain ourselves. We burst out laughing. Red in the face, Dad looked closely at the droppings and realized that they were indeed just brown sprinkles. He studied Mom's gleeful face. Then the look on his face fairly shouted that he had gotten the message. He really needed to enjoy the holiday, lighten up, and declare a temporary truce with the mouse population.

Mary Ann Herlitzke

KEEP AWAY FROM THE WISDOM THAT

DOES NOT CRY,

THE PHILOSOPHY THAT DOES NOT

LAUGH,

AND THE GREATNESS THAT DOES

NOT BOW BEFORE CHILDREN.

Kahlil Gibran

Ask for Help

I was the first elementary guidance counselor in an inner city school in Albany. It was a wonderful job. I loved the students, parents, teachers, and even the court system. Johanne, the principal of the school, was and is a great friend of mine.

We were in the midst of the oil shortage. Oil prices were so high that schools decided to give a longer break at Christmastime. On the Sunday night before the opening of school, Johanne asked me to go with her into the school and turn the heat on so that the students wouldn't be forced to sit all day Monday with their winter coats on.

Snow and ice covered Albany that evening. We parked the car behind the school and entered the ice-cold brick structure. It was freezing in there! The heater was in the basement, so we went down there in order to pull all the appropriate levers and switches.

As we reached the doorway at the top of the basement stairs on our way out, we noticed that the door had slammed shut. Then it hit Johanne. All the locks had been changed over the Christmas vacation. We didn't have a key to get out.

We immediately began thinking of ways we could escape the basement. It was much too cold to remain there all night. We checked the outside cellar door. It wouldn't budge because so much snow had fallen on top of it. There was no way we could force the door open. I placed a chair on the top stair and tried to look out a tiny window. I hoped that someone would walk past the school and we could attract their attention. No one was silly enough to be out in this storm!

Johanne then announced that she had to go to the bathroom. Just the suggestion transferred the same need to me. What would we do? (About a half-hour later as I stayed posted at my window position, I began to hear a trickle coming from the basement. I realized that Johanne had found a drain. This did not help my condition!)

All of a sudden an idea came to me: *pull the fire alarm.* I yelled down to Johanne. Horrified at the idea, she declared that she couldn't do it. "That would bring every fire engine in the city of Albany to the school."

I tried to reason with her. We would freeze if we spent the night in the basement waiting for the heat to activate. No one knew where we were. It didn't seem likely that anyone was going to walk past the school so we could signal for help. "Fire engines even come to get cats out of trees!" I argued. Nothing helped. Johanne could not—would not—pull the handle.

I left my window position and ran down the stairs. Mind you, I was not keen on what I was about to do, I just didn't want to freeze to death and could think of nothing else to do. So I pulled down the red bar on the fire alarm, then ran back up the stairs and resumed my post.

Fire engines arrived from all directions. Lights flashed brilliantly, washing the outside of the school building in red. Then we heard the welcomed footsteps. Several firefighters appeared at the cellar door. As soon as they forced the door open, I ran through. Hurriedly thanking the startled firefighters for rescuing us, I kept moving, saying over my shoulder that I needed to visit the ladies' room before I could explain what happened!

Anyway, I figured Johanne could explain the situation. For months afterward, Johanne and I would regale various audiences—no matter how small—in our version of "The Great Escape." We figured, why let a good story go to waste and, truth be told, the story and our peril grew and grew. But so our own laughter.

THE CREATOR MADE HUMANS ABLE TO WALK AND TALK, TO SEE AND HEAR . . . TO DO EVERYTHING. BUT THE CREATOR WASN'T SATISFIED. FINALLY, THE CREATOR MADE HUMANS LAUGH, AND WHEN THEY LAUGHED AND LAUGHED, THE CREATOR SAID, "NOW YOU ARE FIT TO LIVE."

Traditional Apache Story

WAY 9 :

Pray

PRAYER IS AN ATTITUDE OF THE
HEART THAT CAN TRANSFORM EVERY
ACTIVITY. . . . MOMENTS IN WHICH
WE DRINK DEEPLY FROM THE
SOURCE OF MEANING ARE MOMENTS
OF PRAYER, WHETHER WE CALL
THEM SO OR NOT.

David Steindl-Rast

Any kind of prayer can relieve stress. And prayer helps to heal our emotional, physical, and spiritual ailments. Consider the following study undertaken by a cardiologist at a California hospital: From a group of 393 seriously ill, cardiac patients, 192 were selected randomly for a special treatment. Their conditions were described in detail to people around the country who had been asked to pray for their health and recovery. Five to seven participants were selected to pray daily for each one of these 192 patients. Those praying were asked to focus their prayers on healing and a quick recovery for the patients. The patients were unaware that this study was being done or that people were committed to praying for them. The remaining patients were given quality medical care, but had none of the study's participants praying for them.

Ten months later the people who had been prayed for by others experienced markedly fewer incidences of cardiac-related infections, pulmonary edema, and mortality than did the patients not included. In short, prayer helped healing.

Prayer helps our lives in many ways. When we quiet our minds and become still, wisdom comes to offer us insight, or as a Chinese adage offers, "When the pupil is ready, the teacher will come." Prayer helps us see that there are options, and our perceptual world is broadened. Like humor, prayer relaxes us, giving our minds a chance to become aware that we always have choices. Prayer refreshes our spirits and frees us from the tension we so often hold in our bodies.

An old proverb reminds us: "The winds of grace are blowing perpetually, we only need to raise our sails." Prayer raises the sail of our spirit in full expectation that the winds of grace will push us to safe harbor. At its roots, prayer simply means being aware of the presence of God and our response to that awareness.

The response to the sacred may take many forms. We all pray differently. For some, prayer is formal. Rituals, recitation of specific prayers, singing or chanting holy songs or passages may be clearly defined and structured in group settings. For others, prayer occurs spontaneously in response to the discovery of God in daily happenings. A person may give thanks to the Creator for an awesome sunset, the smile of an elderly person, or the beauty in the face of a child.

Of course, prayer has often been a natural response to distress. Writer John Deedy tells a true story about a fisherman who everyone thought had been lost at sea, drowned in an unexpected storm. Another vessel rescued the man. When a reporter interviewed the survivor, the following interchange took place.

"Were you scared out there, all alone, cold, and wet?" asked the news reporter.

"Yes," replied the seaman.

A bit frustrated by the sailor's failure to elaborate, the reporter probed further. "What did you do out there on the ocean during all those scary hours?"

"I prayed," said the seaman laconically.

"Prayed?" responded the reporter. "What did you pray?"

"Oh, you know. Your basic Our Father and Hail Mary."

When we are scared, lonely, and stressed, we pray any way that we can. This kind of prayer recognizes that we are not in control of the universe. No matter what the form, prayer opens us to the reality that we are part of something bigger than words can ever describe.

Prayer is not a passive behavior, which allows us to make a request and expect that what we ask for will be done. Prayer is an active response or acknowledgment of the presence of the Spirit. It is a way of inviting a sacred friend into our life. The Spirit will support and guide us through the tangled web of stress.

FOR MERCY HAS A HUMAN HEART,

PITY A HUMAN FACE,

AND LOVE, THE HUMAN FORM

DIVINE,

AND PEACE, THE HUMAN DRESS.

THERE EVERY MAN, OF EVERY CLIME,
THAT PRAYS IN HIS DISTRESS,
PRAYS TO THE HUMAN FORM DIVINE,
LOVE, MERCY, PITY, PEACE.

William Blake

Pray

- Create a sacred place. This can be a simple corner of your bedroom with a table, candle, and sacred reading. What you want to create is a quiet, peaceful place in which you can close your eyes and shut out the busyness of the world around you. Then, sit quietly in a chair and close your eyes. Visualize your favorite scene: the ocean, mountains, a stream. Let the peacefulness of that scene come into your body. Then simply speak and listen to the Divine Spirit that dwells inside you.

- Yoga and Tai Chi are wonderful stress remedies. They combine breathing exercises, relaxation techniques, stretching exercises, various physical postures, and meditation that bring new energy into the body. Read a book describing more about Yoga and Tai Chi practices.

- Sit and daydream and wonder at the universe. Appreciate the wonders of nature. In thanks, sing a favorite hymn or song.

- During troubled times, ask for help from God. Pray for a family member or a friend. Speak from your heart, and you will always be heard.

- Offer thanks for the beauty and goodness that surround you.
- As a prayer of gratitude, do a good deed or a random act of kindness.

LIKEWISE THE SPIRIT HELPS US IN
OUR WEAKNESS; FOR WE DO NOT
KNOW HOW TO PRAY AS WE OUGHT,
BUT THAT VERY SPIRIT INTERCEDES
WITH SIGHS TOO DEEP FOR WORDS.

Paul of Tarsus

God Will Provide

A small town became completely submerged because the rainfall was so heavy. The local priest was young and healthy and made every effort to help those who were in difficulties. He waded waist-deep in the water, helping out wherever he could. Some workers came to his assistance in a little boat, but he carried on alone, saying: "God will provide!"

Later, as the water level rose to his chest, another boat came along, and he helped get an elderly woman on board, but refused to go himself. Once again, he intoned with great trust: "God will provide!" Shortly afterward the water was up to his neck, and he had difficulty keeping afloat. This time an air-rescue crew came by in a helicopter and rescued two people to safety from a rooftop. When they tried to get hold of the priest, he insisted they help somebody else as he shouted, "God will provide!"

When they left, the priest eventually was overcome and drowned. Saint Peter met him at the gates of heaven and showed him in to see God. The priest complained bitterly that he'd done everything he could to help others, and yet he himself hadn't been saved. "I put my trust in you, God," he said. "Why didn't you do anything?"

"What do you mean I didn't do anything?" replied God. "Didn't I send you two boats and a helicopter!"

Prayer often offers us new ways of dealing with situations. But it may come in answers we don't expect or in a manner foreign to us. We can rely on God providing, but the providing often comes from human hands inspired by God.

PRAYER INDEED IS GOOD BUT WHILE CALLING ON THE GODS A MAN SHOULD LEND HIMSELF A HAND.

Hippocrates

Into Your Hands

Since Gene had moved to San Francisco, we had not seen each other in quite a while. So I felt a special lightness as I walked into the Chinese restaurant.

Though I relished the thought of delectable prawns, succulent egg rolls, and sizzling rice soup, I mostly wanted this time to catch up with my friend, indeed one of my oldest, dearest friends. I knew that he had gone through hard times with his marriage. I was about to find out just how hard.

Gene spotted me as I approached the table, stood up quickly—almost pulling the tablecloth off—and wrapped me in his best bear hug. This kind of exuberant affection had always been one of the things I most enjoyed about Gene. Standing 6'4" and weighing nearly 270 pounds, Gene outweighed a lot of bears, but inside the man beat one of the kindest, wisest hearts that I had ever encountered. I noticed that some other diners were gaping at the two of us, but I couldn't have cared less.

After we ordered, I didn't want to waste time beating around the bush, so I asked, "Okay, ol' friend, what's been going on with you and Sharon? The last time we talked, you sounded at the end of the line."

"Well, you know that we've been having hard times. Not exactly 'we.' We haven't been 'we' in years. And I just couldn't take it anymore, kids or no kids."

Gene had met Sharon twenty years before. He was working his way through college as an orderly in a hospital. Some years older than Gene, Sharon had been a nurse on a floor he frequently worked on. She was steady, stable, and never seemed to get too worked up about anything. Gene, on the other hand, came from a crazy family and overflowed with emotions he did not always know what to do with. While many of us never warmed to Sharon, Gene loved her. We wondered how such a warm—somewhat wild—guy like Gene would adjust to a relationship with someone almost the opposite. For some years, it seemed to work.

Over the years, Gene developed a national reputation as a business consultant. He traveled all over, teaching managers how to do strategic planning and build morale among employees. He also discovered that he was funny. His wacky humor and understanding of human nature combined in presentations that broke ice and helped uptight executives talk about the hard issues. And Gene began to appreciate the intuitive and spontaneous facets of his character.

Unfortunately, as Gene's world expanded, Sharon's world contracted. Once Gene's salary could support the family, Sharon announced that she wanted to quit nursing and stay at home with their three children. That had been a dozen years ago. During those years, Gene realized that Sharon did not really have any friends. She never went out, except to school functions. Her world revolved around feeding the kids, keeping house, and rooting for the San Francisco 49ers. While she dutifully asked him about his work, Gene recognized the blank stare he got back as he talked about the people he had met and the places he had gone.

"We stopped sleeping together a bunch of years ago. I might as well have a vow of chastity. I realized one night that I had been fooling myself all those years. We hadn't been making love. She wanted kids. Sex was the way you got kids. When we had our three, it became all too obvious, she just didn't care anymore. I could stand that, though, easier than her blank looks and narrow world. I swear I encouraged her to get updated and licensed to nurse again. I told her if she didn't want to do that then go back to school for something else. She just didn't want to. She'd smile and say, 'I'll think about it.' But nothing ever happened. Do you know how terrifying it is to realize that the woman you loved can only talk with any enthusiasm about a damn football team?"

Gene survived emotionally off the energy he got giving conferences and working. Being on the road meant that he didn't have to face Sharon's blank gazes and lack of affection and engagement. Being on the road also meant that Gene met bright, capable, charming women who found him attractive, interesting, and desirable. Gene confessed that he got so angry with Sharon that he was seriously tempted. Always though, he hoped that somehow his relationship with Sharon could turn around. And, there were his kids. No matter how bad things got with Sharon, he wanted to protect the kids.

"Finally, I suggested to Sharon that we needed counseling. You know what her response was, 'Well, if you want me to go with you so you can talk about your problems, you know I will, Gene.' She had no clue or was in denial, I don't know.

"Anyway, that was the last straw. I felt hopeless. I started waking up in the middle of the night angry. I'd been having a hard time sleeping before, but now it was every night. What was I going to do? What about the kids? What would happen to Sharon if we got a divorce? Who would get the house? On and on. Next thing I'd find myself sitting in the kitchen crying.

"I decided I needed some counseling even if Sharon wouldn't go. That helped some, but the real source of help came in another way. You know I've always gone to church on Sunday. Well I went on Good Friday, and here I was sitting with Sharon and the kids when the reader read Jesus' words from the cross, 'Into your hands I commend my spirit.' It was like the first time I ever heard these words. I sat there stunned.

"Anyway, from then on, when I woke up in the middle of the night and found myself in the kitchen, I started praying, 'God, into your hands I commend my spirit.' Over and over I'd pray it. Pretty soon I would go back to bed and sleep like a rock. During the next few months, real gradually, I didn't even have to get out of bed. When I woke up, I'd just start praying those words and soon I'd go back to sleep. Then during the day when something would make me think and get ticked off at Sharon I'd say my prayer, and I'd be okay."

After our lunch together, contact with Gene again diminished. Then about three years later when his last child left for college, I heard he filed for divorce. The three years of waiting had given him time to work out the practical matters and had given time for the children to gain their own strength.

Gene mailed me a Christmas card shortly after. "Well, amigo," Gene wrote, "I don't know what the future holds. Maybe the right woman will come into my life. I'm okay, though, about that. After all these years of 'commending my spirit' at least I feel much more at peace."

LET NOTHING UPSET YOU,

LET NOTHING AFFRIGHT YOU,

EVERYTHING IS CHANGING;

GOD ALONE IS CHANGELESS.

PATIENCE ATTAINS THE GOAL.
WHO HAS GOD LACKS NOTHING;
GOD ALONE FILLS ALL HER NEEDS.

Teresa of Avila

WAY 10:

Let Go of Negative Baggage

A WISE MAN SEES AS MUCH AS HE
OUGHT, NOT AS MUCH AS HE CAN.

Montaigne

Holding on to old hurts, angers, and disappointments keeps us stuck in a wringer of stress, worry, and fear. We need to pack these away and choose to live in the present moment that is filled with the grace we need. The weight of this negative baggage slumps our shoulders and shrivels our spirits. Unfortunately, though, we can carry this baggage almost unconsciously. We get caught walking in a rut with it and, as an acquaintance always remarks, "The only difference between a rut and a grave is the depth."

Everyone has people reminding them of something they used to do or something that occurred several years back. All of us need to let go and move on. If we stay put we will wither up and die.

Old baggage blocks our perceptions and blinds us to ways we could move on. It will eventually get in the way of our personal goals. These dark perceptions cause disruptions with family members and colleagues and prevent our relationships from being whole and wholesome. We tend to limit our own personal growth and we get tired out.

When we let go of our old stuff, we see where our real power and freedom reside. We are called to flower, grow, and become. Life is a process of continually opening up ourselves to what is and what can be. To hold on to what was is a dead end street. No one can change yesterday. We cannot take a thing back that we said or change a thing we did. All we can do is begin each day anew.

Letting go of old arguments, ancient hurts, and bitter stories takes conscious effort. Our spirits tend to keep track of negative baggage like tourists guarding their suitcases and golf bags in a busy airport. Unlike the tourists, our journey through life would be much more enjoyable without having to drag all this garbage along with us. But, we must look at all the baggage, name it, claim it, decide we don't need it anymore, and then dump it. Mark Twain offers us this advice: "Drag your thoughts away from your troubles—by the ears, by the heels, or any other way you can manage. It's the healthiest thing a body can do."

ONE OF THE THINGS I LEARNED THE HARD WAY WAS THAT IT DOESN'T PAY TO GET DISCOURAGED. KEEPING BUSY AND MAKING OPTIMISM A WAY OF LIFE CAN RESTORE YOUR FAITH IN YOURSELF.

Lucille Ball

Let Go of Negative Baggage

- Learn to track your own thoughts. Listen to yourself. Don't suppress your thoughts. Let them come, run their course, and then let them go. We tend to give them too much power if we hold on to them.

- Tell someone about the negative baggage you are carrying inside of you. On the other hand, do not tell everyone you meet about your problems from the past. If you do, you are only rehearsing the situation and no resolution ever comes from that. If you find yourself returning to the negative stuff over and over with this confidant, consider talking with a professional counselor.

- Know when to get help. The healthy person can ask for what is needed. Your stress level can build up to an unhealthy level, and then you may have to see a mental health professional to help you deal with your stress and fears. Reach out to your minister, priest, or rabbi if you are not in a position to go to a therapist.

- Tell yourself good things about yourself. Sometimes we can't get out of a rut because we push ourselves down so far, remembering the mistakes we've made or the things that have not worked out the way we think they should have. Affirming yourself becomes a healthy way of keeping balance in your own life. Write out a list of self-affirmations. Focus on gifts, talents, abilities, and qualities of character. Recite one of these regularly for a week, then use another the next week and the next.

- When we carry old angers or old hurts inside, the only ones that are burdened with the weight of those are us—the ones holding on to them. We can let go of those angers and hurts by writing unsent letters to those people to whom we need to say things. Address the unsent letter to the person, and then write and write and write—spelling and punctuation don't count! What is important is that we write all our thoughts and feelings, and consequently, release those angers and hurts. After we are finished writing the letter, it helps to reread it. We will be surprised at our handwriting. We may also be surprised at what we wrote. Then perform a letting go ritual: tear the letter up in a million little pieces or burn the letter piece by piece. As you tear or burn, say something like this: "With this act I let go of this painful time. I free myself for new life." What is important is that we have written the letter and have let the feelings go. The goal is to get rid of that ache and not have it part of our life any more.

WE ARE NEVER HAPPY FOR A
THOUSAND DAYS,
A FLOWER NEVER BLOOMS FOR A
HUNDRED.

Chinese Proverb

Playing Santa

One Christmas season I went with the Telephone Pioneers, a service organization sponsored by the New York State Telephone Company, to New York City to play Santa Claus. The eighty of us climbed on two buses to begin our trip to the City. Once on the New York Thruway the buses stopped at a rest area, and we were each given a Santa suit. We were instructed to begin putting them on since we wouldn't have enough time once we went through Lincoln Tunnel.

Each of us made an agreement with the Telephone Pioneers to go wherever we were asked to go. It could have been a hospital, a prison, or an orphanage. It really didn't matter to me. I relished the chance to be Santa.

Once we arrived in the city we were told that we were going to Metropolitan Hospital in Harlem. As we walked into the lobby of the hospital, smiles greeted us. Young children stood in awe. No one wondered out loud that there were eighty of us Santas.

The hospital representative came to greet us and asked if some of us would be willing to go to the psychiatric unit. I was a natural, and so volunteered. Since there were so many of us Santas, we were sent in groups of four to each unit. I was assigned the adolescent unit.

As they unlocked the doors, we could hear the teens' loud music and saw several of them in various positions of relaxation lounging around the room.

I walked around, talking to several of the patients, and then noticed a young girl on the other side of the room standing by herself. She was dressed in hospital attire, which would indicate that she had not been on the unit for long.

I walked over to her. "How long have you been here?"

"I came yesterday."

"Wow, how scary for you. You don't know the routine around here. I bet you don't even know many people's names."

She nodded, then she sat down. I sat in the chair right next to her. We continued our conversation.

"What's your name?"

"Victoria," she responded.

"What a beautiful name." And a beautiful smile appeared on her face.

"What a gorgeous smile you have."

The smile vanished from her face.

"Victoria, why did you stop smiling? Smiling can help you. Smiles help us feel better."

Victoria looked at me and began talking. She told me about her family and the difficulties that lead her to this hospital. In our ten-minute conversation, Victoria shared much about her fourteen years of life. Again, a beautiful smile came to her face.

"Victoria, you must keep smiling. Even if you don't feel like doing it, smiling makes you feel better."

"I never knew that." Then, she quickly got up from the chair and walked away.

I was there to interact with the adolescents, and so I turned to meet Nicole, a slightly younger girl who was standing nearby.

She was a talkative eleven-year-old who seemed to share every thought she ever had with me. Nicole had been in the unit for two months and knew the routine. It was apparent that she enjoyed talking to this Santa. She asked about my reindeer and the snow in the North Pole. Then she asked if I would like to see a bulletin board that was made with my sleigh and reindeer on it. I knew she was joshing a bit about her "belief" in Santa, but I played along.

She took me to another section of the unit where I saw the bulletin board. I paused in delight and called each of the reindeer by name. I was grateful that we sang "Rudolph the Red-Nosed Reindeer" while we were on the bus. It brought back all the reindeer names to me.

Before I left Nicole I asked her what type of behavior she was trying to correct before she could be discharged from the unit.

Without a second's hesitation she said, "I have to stop trying to kill myself."

"Nicole, I need you to promise me that you will never try to kill yourself again."

Instantly she promised me. But I needed to continue. "No, you can't make a promise that quickly. And never make a promise to Santa unless you plan on keeping it. Nicole, I want you to get up every morning and say, 'I am a good person. I am going to take care of myself. I am going to like myself.'"

Nicole looked at me with her beautiful brown eyes and repeated those words somewhat quietly to me. Then I got one of the warmest hugs I have ever gotten in my life.

At that moment we heard the announcement over the address system of the hospital. "Calling all Santas. Please meet on the bus immediately."

We had to leave. My body walked away, but my heart and mind stayed with them. I got on the bus and wondered why we couldn't stay there all day. We went to have lunch and joined other Santas in the New York City Christmas Parade. I returned to Albany that night with Nicole and Victoria in my heart. Perhaps a few minutes with Santa would touch their hearts. Maybe Santa did leave some gifts when she helped carry away their switches and ashes.

DON'T CARRY A GRUDGE. WHILE
YOU'RE CARRYING A GRUDGE,
THE OTHER GUY IS OUT DANCING.

Buddy Hackett

The Wrong Luggage

I had just given a conference in Dubuque, Iowa. My plane had to stop in La Crosse, Wisconsin, on the way to Chicago. This small plane required us to place our carry-on suitcases outside the plane and get a ticket. When we landed, we would then retrieve our suitcase and take them on our next plane.

As we arrived at Chicago's O'Hare, I noticed that our suitcases were lined up along the side of the plane, and that there were a few identical bags. I was the last person to depart the plane. Only one bag awaited me. It looked like my suitcase except that it had a lock on it. Mine didn't.

I asked the baggage handler what to do. He said that I could go into the airport and have the person behind the counter page the owner of this bag. The call went out: "Robert Martin, Robert Martin. Please return to G-8. Robert Martin. Please return to G-8."

About ten minutes later, I went up to the counter and asked her if she could repeat the page. This time she sent the page over to the K and H terminals too. She looked up Robert Martin on the computer and told me that he was going to Fort Lauderdale and that his plane was leaving at 5:30 from Gate H-1, a different terminal. It was only 3:30, but my plane was leaving for Albany at 4:30.

I began my walk over to the H terminal. Of course, Chicago's O'Hare Airport is huge. I stopped in every store, bar, shoeshine booth, and restaurant that I passed. I walked my entire journey looking at the floor for a suitcase that looked like mine. Occasionally I'd even yell out, "Robert Martin! Robert Martin!"

Arriving at H-1, I went over to the ticket counter and asked the gentleman if he would page Robert Martin. I explained my situation to him. He graciously tried to help. "If Robert Martin is sitting in the waiting area, would he please come over to the counter immediately." I waited. No Robert Martin.

Looking at my watch and realizing that I would miss my plane unless I got back to my own gate, I turned to begin the trek back. As I passed a group of about five men I heard one say, "They keep paging Martin. Wonder what they want him for."

I swung around and said, "Do you know Robert Martin? I'm looking for him because he has my suitcase. My car keys are in it."

One of the men said that Robert Martin was up in the VIP lounge. Rushing back to the H-1 counter, I requested that they call the VIP lounge and ask Robert Martin to bring me my luggage. Not yet hopeless, I began my trip back. I reminded myself of all the stress principles I teach others. "What's the worst possible thing that will happen? My luggage will arrive a day late. As far as the car keys being in the suitcase, I do know a few people in Albany I could call to get a ride home."

I was almost back at my departure gate when I saw a man walking quite quickly past me, pulling my suitcase.

"Robert Martin?" I yelled. He stopped dead. I continued, "You picked up my suitcase by mistake. It looks just like yours, but you have a lock and I don't." At that point the employees behind the counter noticed I found my suitcase and started to cheer.

Mr. Martin began explaining what happened. I stopped him and said, "Mistakes happen. No problem. I just wanted my suitcase back because my car keys were in it."

Still, Mr. Martin was defensive. "I didn't take your suitcase on purpose and I didn't take anything out of it," he shot back. "I never even opened it. You check right now in front of all these people from the airlines. You'll see. I didn't take a thing."

I said that wouldn't be necessary. I was not accusing him of taking anything. I also joked, "You would have been surprised if you had opened my suitcase and found only my dirty laundry!"

Flying home that afternoon I felt sad. Sad that Mr. Martin would immediately think I didn't trust him. I wondered what experiences occurred in his life that triggered that response from him. I wondered what baggage—not luggage, but psychological baggage—he needed to let go of. Who didn't trust him? How was he judged in the past? How did he become distrustful of others? He found his own suitcase, but I felt sure that it was not as heavy as his negative emotional baggage.

THE ONLY PLACE OUTSIDE HEAVEN
WHERE YOU CAN BE PERFECTLY
SAFE FROM ALL THE DANGERS OF
LOVE . . . IS HELL.

C. S. Lewis

WAY 11 :

Just Say "No"

SAYING NO CAN BE THE ULTIMATE
SELF-CARE.

Claudia Black

In this time of downsizing, companies are trying to do more with less money and fewer employees. As a result, workers are pressured into more overtime with higher expectations from management. Some job stresses come from not knowing what shift you may be working, being "on call" during off hours, being expected to work overtime, and not taking deserved vacation time. Policies seem to change constantly. Job objectives are kept murky. Time pressures and deadlines squeeze us. And job security has vanished in the dot com age.

If we want to kick the stress habit, many of us have to learn to say a simple word, "no." We must take control of our own calendars. Saying "no" to some meetings or other demands on our time can help us reduce stress. We must remember that it is impossible to complete everything at once. When "no" is an appropriate response, it frees the speaker and releases pressure.

Some of us have difficulty saying "no" because we are afraid others won't like us. Yet as mythologist Joseph Campbell pointed out, "Jesus said love your enemies, he didn't say don't have any."

Some believe that saying "no" is selfish and rude, but saying "yes" when you want to say "no" decreases your self-confidence and self-esteem. People who have to say "yes" build up a lot of resentment and frustration toward others. After a while they get tired of putting other people first. Chronic "yes" people begin to think everyone else is more important. This negatively affects relationships. They begin dreading being with people who seem to disrespect their time and only fulfill their needs. Feeling that they are out of control and always pleasing everyone else catches up with them, and they want to avoid being with these demanding people.

Strangely, most people can accept the response of an honest "no." Most people understand that others have needs and responsibilities and that there are times when the needs of others cannot be put aside. What is important is for us to be in charge of the person we see in the mirror. We have to know our own needs and believe that we are worthwhile persons. We have the right to create limits for our own time.

"No" is hard to say sometimes. People-pleasers would rather hide. But to constantly put the needs of others in front of our own needs creates high levels of stress and anxiety. After all, who wants to stay in the company of someone who disregards our needs or treats us like a gofer?

The hardest part of learning the art of saying "no" is doing it for the first time. Initially we almost choke on the word. We anticipate the worst and expect outrage from the person making the request. What a surprise when the other person can accept our "no."

In learning to say "no," three guidelines can help. First, try to be brief and quick with your response. To hesitate or to ramble on often sends a message of uncertainty. When you know that you need to say "no," do so with security.

Second, if you believe that sometime in the future you might be interested in accepting the invitation or taking part in the activity, simply tell the other person something like this: "Thank you for thinking of me for this, but I cannot do it presently. If sometime in the future it comes up again, please feel free to ask me again." Or, "No, I won't be able to meet you for lunch on Monday. But thank you for asking me." You are saying a firm "no" but not burning any bridges.

The third guideline is to separate the request from the person. It may be difficult to say "no" to someone you love, are afraid of, or are dependent on, but you have to keep in mind that you are responding to the request and not rejecting the person.

LET YOUR "YES" BE YES AND YOUR "NO" BE NO.

Letter of James

Just Say "No"

- Stand in front of a mirror and look yourself in the eye. Say the word "no" softly. Repeat that five more times. Now say the word a bit louder. Repeat that five more times. If you feel resistance while saying "no," keep practicing until it becomes a fixed part of your vocabulary.

- Recall a time when "no" was your response. What happened? Were there any serious repercussions? any repercussions at all?

- Besides saying "no" to others, it is also important to say "no" to ourselves. For example:
  - "no" to that extra piece of chocolate candy
  - "no" to another drink
  - "no" to putting our whole paycheck on a bet.

- Gentle, persistent repeating of your "no" is also very effective. For example:
  - "No, you can't go to the shopping mall." When the child pleads again, simply repeat in a moderate, calm tone of voice, "No, you cannot go to the shopping mall." (This repeating of a simple phrase is a technique that is called The Broken Record.)

- Recall some instances in the recent past in which you said "yes" when you really wanted to say a firm "no." Think about the extra hassles your response caused you.

May those who love us, love us.

And may those who don't love us,

May God turn their hearts.

And if God doesn't turn their

HEARTS

MAY HE TURN THEIR ANKLES,

SO WE WILL KNOW THEM BY THEIR

LIMPING.

Traditional Celtic Lore

Ski Trip

"**I** regretted my decision as soon as my daughter walked out the door that night," Don Burlingame, parent of fifteen-year-old Amanda, recalled a few days after he gave Amanda permission to go on a Friday night ski trip to a local resort with her friends.

Amanda was a good skier; Don had taught her himself.

Amanda had been on many ski outings without Don or her mom, Laura, before, but those were always with the official school ski club, with adult drivers and chaperones from the faculty at the high school.

Amanda was also exemplary as a person; she was an "A" student who was active in her church youth group. Don knew she was not a "party girl" and did not worry about her or her friends—sixteen-year-olds Roy and Meg, and fifteen-year-old Josh—drinking or doing anything else illegal while they were out.

"Still, after I watched from the window as they pulled away, I had an uneasy sense about my decision. Though I trusted Amanda and her friends to make good decisions, I couldn't help but think of all the other kooks that would be out on the road and on the slopes on a Friday night."

Don explained how Amanda had originally asked if she could go. "She worked on her mom first. Laura's kind of smitten herself over Amanda's friend Josh. I think Amanda and Laura both thought of this as a kind of non-threatening first date.

"By the time they approached me on Monday night I was easy pickins. It seemed like I had no choice."

The group of skiers pulled out of Don's driveway at 6:30. Amanda was to call when they arrived at the resort, about a twenty-mile drive. She was also to call when they were on their way home at the agreed upon 11 p.m. closing time. All that went off as planned.

"When the clock struck midnight and my daughter wasn't home yet I imagined the worst," said Don.

The next call came at 12:17. By that time Don and Laura were at their wits' end with worry. A state trooper identified himself.

"Mr. Burlingame, there has been an accident. Everyone is okay," the voice announced.

Though the man spoke his entire message as if one sentence, Don only heard the first part: accident. He felt a mixture of fear, anger, and regret come over him. Mainly he was overwhelmed by the love he had for his daughter. He had to get to her.

When Don and Laura arrived at the scene, just ten minutes from their house, two sights greeted them simultaneously: One was Roy's sports utility vehicle laying on its side in the ditch by the side of the road. The other was Amanda, with tears in her eyes but otherwise all together, running up to her mom for a hug.

A deer had run across the road, Roy swerved away, and the car ended up on its side. None of the kids was injured seriously. Amanda's only pain came from when she fell slightly after releasing her seatbelt when the car came to a stop.

Don reflected on the incident a few days later. "I know I can't overprotect my daughter. She has to have some freedom to make choices for her own life. On the other hand she's still legally, morally, and emotionally my responsibility. The next time something doesn't feel just right, I think I will exercise my father prerogative and say 'no.'"

Michael Maestas

I CAN'T GIVE YOU THE FORMULA
FOR SUCCESS. I CAN FOR FAILURE:
TRY TO PLEASE EVERYONE.

Bill Cosby

Crossing New Territory

Working all summer in the Ozark Mountains of Arkansas made me the envy of many of my high school classmates. This was my second summer as a counselor at the Boy Scout camp. I loved canoeing, swimming, and best of all, teaching younger kids all that I had learned about scouting. And I was good at it. The chief reason that I later became a teacher was because of my success as a counselor at camp. But it might have all been different without what I know now was a crucial time in my life.

I was seventeen, but had been hired as the assistant program director of the camp. Terry, the program director, was twenty-five, and most of the other staff members were university students. Being in this position gave me a tremendous shot of confidence, but being younger than the other guys I was directing sometimes left me feeling pretty insecure. Several of the older guys were none too happy that I had been chosen over them. Most respected me and worked well with me. Even so, I had doubts about myself.

One day in July, two scoutmasters asked me to lead their boys on a five-mile cross-country hike to the outpost camp. I wasn't too sure that this was a good idea. I showed them the route on a topographical map. It took us across a series of steep ridges and a lot of rough terrain. I expressed my doubts about the ability of the younger kids to do such a strenuous workout. They persisted. I kept discouraging them. Finally, somewhat angered by my reluctance, they told the program director that they wanted to go and that he should order me to lead them.

Terry simply said, "Ah, go ahead. It's their funeral." I thought that it might not be a funeral, but it sure could be an extremely unpleasant experience for some of the kids.

The next day we departed right after lunch. As we headed into the woods, I noticed that many of the kids wore shorts—something that I had discouraged because of poison ivy and a whole variety of other creeping and crawling things—and many had no canteen—something else that I had insisted on. I held my anger inside, figuring that the adults were responsible and should have known better.

The first three miles went well enough. The terrain was every bit as rough as I had told them and the hills as steep, but the kids slogged on. We stopped for a break on a promontory overlooking a bend in the Spring River. The green hills and meadows stretched out for miles. The sound of the river bubbling over rapids drifted up from below us.

"Carl, I've got two kids with terrible poison ivy. They're in bad shape. What are you going to do?" The scoutmaster's face was red from the sun and from his anger. It was directed at me. I bit back a smart retort.

I looked at the two kids. Neither wore long pants, both were covered with poison ivy's red welts. They had to be terribly allergic to be in this kind of trouble so quickly.

The two scoutmasters continued to harp at me. "You never told us that we would be hiking through all this crap. These kids have to get back and see the doctor. There's a road down there. Let's take it, and we'll make better time." Still I refrained from arguing. My guts churned from anger, fear, and guilt.

I pulled out the topographical map and showed them that the road might look easier, but would actually add three miles to our hike. Where we stood was just less than two miles from the outpost. "Besides," I said, "the terrain between here and the outpost levels out and should be smoother sailing."

They would have none of it. "Well, we're the scoutmasters, and we're going to take the kids on the road." With that they told the kids that they were going to climb down the bluffs and take the road. The kids looked from them to me, wondering who was right. Finally, feeling defeated, I nodded. "Okay, let's go."

The rest of the trek became more of a nightmare. To get to the road, we had to cross the river. All of us got our feet wet, which meant that we walked in soggy shoes the rest of the way. The kids soldiered on for the first couple of miles but soon began dragging. When we came to the first house, the scoutmasters hired the farmer to haul the younger kids to the base camp in his truck. The rest of us, silent and exhausted, walked into the outpost camp just after sunset.

I heard the scoutmasters telling the outpost director about how stupid I was, how I should have known better than to take this hike, and so on. Fortunately, I knew Buzz well. He had a general disdain for the type of adult who would blame a teenager for their mistakes. Buzz just listened silently.

The outpost staff made room for the new troop, helped them get cleaned up, and fed them. I hid out with a couple of my staff buddies who listened to my side of the story. They were sympathetic, but I felt sick at my acquiescence, at my waffling and weakness. And I dreaded the sure confrontation with the director when we returned to the main camp the next day.

After we returned, I got word that the camp director, Mr. Young, wanted to see me. Fearful and ashamed, I entered his office.

"Mr. Young, I. . . ." He cut me off.

"Carl, I just have two things to say. First, those two men are adults. The responsibility rests on them a lot more than it does on you. Second, the last two summers you've shown yourself to be smart, capable, and responsible, but"—he paused and looked me square in the face—"you have to trust yourself more. Listen to your own good judgment. Don't let people who don't know what the hell is going on shove you around. Have more confidence in yourself. Now get back to work and forget this."

Mr. Young gave me a priceless gift that day. Since then, I have learned to let my "no" be "no" and my "yes" be "yes." Sure I've made mistakes since—lots of them—but they have been my mistakes and my triumphs too.

Carl Koch

SELF-RESPECT IS THE FRUIT OF DIS-CIPLINE, THE SENSE OF DIGNITY GROWS WITH THE ABILITY TO SAY NO TO ONESELF.

Abraham Heschel

Be Grateful, Give Thanks

GRATITUDE TAKES THREE FORMS:

A FEELING IN THE HEART,

AN EXPRESSION IN WORDS,

AND A GIVING IN RETURN.

Proverbs

A wise old man was resting on the side of a road. A traveler approached and asked if he knew what the people were like in the town ahead. The wise old man asked, "What were the people like in the town you just came from?" The traveler replied, "Oh, they were nasty and rude. I couldn't trust anyone." The wise old man told him that the people in the town ahead were the same.

A bit later another traveler stopped to ask the wise old man about the people in the town ahead. The wise man responded again by asking the traveler what the people were like in the town he just came from. The traveler replied, "Oh, they were caring, warm, wonderful people." And the wise old man told the traveler that the people in the town up ahead were exactly the same.

The moral of the story is: Things are not as they are, but as we are. If we readily appreciate the goodness in life and the beauty that surrounds us, we nourish a good heart within ourselves and a grateful spirit that generously gives thanks. Upon honest reflection, we have many more reasons to give thanks than to worry. Gratitude and thankfulness dispel stress and banish worry. Now science supports what wisdom has suggested for centuries.

Recent scientific research indicates that positive emotions such as gratitude and love have beneficial effects on health. Positive emotions strengthen and enhance the immune system, which enables the body to resist disease and recover more quickly from illness. Endorphins, the body's natural painkillers, are released into the bloodstream and they stimulate dilation of the blood vessels, which leads to a relaxed heart, among other effects.

Negative emotions such as anger, worry, and hopelessness reduce the number of endorphins and slow the movement of disease-fighting white cells in our bloodstream. By dumping high levels of adrenaline into the bloodstream, negative emotions contribute to the development of stroke and heart disease. Adrenaline constricts the blood vessels, particularly to the heart, raising blood pressure and potentially damaging arteries and the heart itself.

On the other hand, when we count our blessings we shower our bodies with health. Counting our blessings helps us focus on the wonders of life. A thankful spirit chooses to look at what is right in our lives rather than the negative. Counting our blessings opens us to actually see what is right in front of us, the vast array of which is good and true.

A few years ago I was privileged to hear renowned psychiatrist Victor Frankl give a keynote address. Frankl was a survivor of the concentration camp at Auschwitz. He told the audience that he would never have made it if he could not have laughed: "It lifted me momentarily out of this horrible situation, just enough to make it livable. . . . We who lived in concentration camps can remember the men who walked through the huts comforting others, giving away their last piece of bread. They may have been few in number, but they offer sufficient proof that everything can be taken from a man but one thing: the last of the human freedoms— to choose one's attitude in any given set of circumstances." He knew that cursing life can kill us; being thankful and grateful keeps the spirit alive.

Counting our blessings is not often encouraged and is frequently put down. However, counting blessings means focusing on the positive: to see that the rain helps vegetables grow, the long line at the grocery store gives me a few silent moments for myself, the drive to work allows me to savor every moment and let the hurried person pass me. Having a grateful heart offers the opportunity to give my colleagues praise and energy, to see that employers are human and I am responsible only for how I act.

There is a marvelous story about the famous Berlin Wall. I've heard a few variations of the story. The essence is the same.

Emotions were high-pitched in Berlin in the early days of the infamous Berlin Wall. Hostilities flared when those living in the eastern sector dumped truckloads of stinking garbage over the wall into West Berlin. Mayor Willie Brandt was flooded with demands for revenge at this offense.

Brandt responded in a unique way. He requested that every flower in West Berlin be brought to a specific place at the wall. Then, as a great avalanche of fragrant and beautiful flowers was poured over the wall into East Berlin, a large banner was raised. Written on the banner were the words, "We each give what we have."

Giving thanks and words of gratitude to one another, to God, and to the universe gladden our heart, vanquish stress, and make us healthy. So, be grateful, give thanks.

FEAR LESS, HOPE MORE, EAT LESS,

CHEW MORE, WHINE LESS, BREATHE

MORE, TALK LESS,

SAY MORE, LOVE MORE, AND

ALL GOOD THINGS WILL BE YOURS.

Swedish Proverb

Be Grateful, Give Thanks

- Write a short, hand-written note to someone, telling them how grateful you are for something they did for you. Mail the note.

- Call a friend or family member and thank them for being a part of your life.

- Keep a Blessings-of-the-Day log. Every day, write down at least three blessings. Allow yourself to be surprised. Let yourself stop long enough to remember a small kindness, or notice some surprise of nature: the first snow of winter, the first buds of spring, or a sunset. Surprise is the beginning of gratefulness, a kind of rousing that we may need to get accustomed to as a gradual way into gratitude.

- Or, if you prefer, right after you crawl into bed for the night, tell your spouse if you have one or God if you don't about several things for which you are grateful for from your day. Ending the day recalling blessings can ease our stress and smooth our way into sleep.

- Spend a few minutes looking out at nature. Breathe in the fresh air. Feel the freshness of the season. Let the beauty of the moment come into your heart and soul.

- Think of five things that happened to you over your lifetime that brought joy and happiness to you. Be grateful for those things. Whenever you are tempted to gloom, remember these occasions.

- Remember a time when someone thanked you for something you did. How did that make you feel?

- Every night, when you crawl into bed, recall the blessings of the day: "What am I grateful for today?"

GRATITUDE IS NOT ONLY THE
GREATEST OF ALL THE VIRTUES, BUT
THE PARENT OF ALL THE OTHERS.

Cicero

Taxi

Recently I was picked up at Islip Airport on Long Island. The driver had frustration written all over his face when he rolled down the passenger window and questioned, "Sister Anne?" I said, "Yes." He motioned with his thumb for me to get into the back seat of the cab.

The driver nervously smoked a cigarette. Cigarette smoke really bothers me. My head gets filled, my eyes water, and I have a hard time breathing. He asked me where I was going, and I immediately told him the name of the country club where I was to speak. He asked if I had ever been there before. I said I had.

"Good. Tell me how to get there. I don't know where it is."

I told him that I was not familiar with Long Island. He began puffing his cigarette more intently and picked up a spiral book that contained detail maps. He frantically turned pages and then threw the book back down on the seat. He announced that he needed gas and that so far the day had been a disaster. He had just left LaGuardia Airport where he was supposed to deliver a package, but no one would sign for it.

He went for gas and then picked up his CB, asked for directions, and was told he could find the country club on Jerioke Turnpike in Woodbury in the red section of his map book. As we began our adventure of finding Woodbury, I asked him if he had been in this business a long time. He told me that he had, but hated it because the company he worked for was "terrible."

"You shouldn't stay in it," I offered. "Life is too short."

He said he had no choice. Then we stopped for a red light. In the rear window of the van that had stopped in front of us, a sign read: "Drivers wanted—full-time and part-time."

I quickly said, "There's a sign saying they need drivers. Take down that number."

"That company is worse than this one."

Just then a car pulled around another and cut in front of us. Annoyed, I said, "People don't have any patience."

"No patience. No caring. No compassion."

Silently we continued on the Long Island Expressway. Finally, I asked, "Are you married?"

"No."

A long period of silence followed. Then he said, "I grew up in the Bronx. When people find out you don't have a mother or father, they don't want you to go out with their daughter. Funny, though, they can abuse their daughters." I tried to respond to his hurt and rejection. He told me he was through looking for a woman to marry.

When I got out of the car, I felt sad. Here was a lonely young man trapped in negativity. He held on to the fact that he had no parents, really had no one who cared about him, and that was the way it would always be. No one would get to see a caring, compassionate, grateful person. He was going to stay guarded and invulnerable.

My driver that day was focusing on what he didn't have. All the while, he had good health. He received a paycheck each month. He had a house. Sadly, he did not know how to be grateful and thankful for what he *did* have. For him life would continue to be undeliverable packages, lack of direction, and an empty tank.

The taxi driver filled with sadness put me in mind of the father of my friend Sister Roselani. I was privileged to have met Toshi Enomoto at his home in Maui, Hawaii. Toshi was a wise man who greeted his visitors with a smile of hospitality. When anyone asked him how he was, Toshi always gave the same quick response, "More grateful than ever." He did not dwell on his inability to get around, his loss of hearing, and the deaths of his wife and loved ones. Toshi had learned the secret of being happy. He had chosen to be grateful for what he had and the blessings that had graced his life.

More grateful than ever.

IN THE EVENING, WHEN I LIE IN BED AND END MY PRAYERS WITH THE WORDS, "I THANK YOU, GOD, FOR ALL THAT IS GOOD AND DEAR AND BEAUTIFUL," I AM FILLED WITH JOY. . . . I DON'T THINK THEN OF ALL THE MISERY, BUT OF THE BEAUTY THAT STILL REMAINS. . . . LOOK AT THESE THINGS, THEN YOU FIND YOURSELF AGAIN, AND GOD, AND THEN YOU REGAIN YOUR BALANCE.

Anne Frank

Loretta

When the phone rings in the evening around suppertime, I grimace. Usually some telemarketer wants to send me a new credit card or offer a special deal on a time-share unit in the Wisconsin Dells. My wife and I look at the phone, each of us hating to pick it up. We do though. Mostly because this is my mother-in-law Loretta's favorite time to call too.

As soon as I picked up the phone, Loretta blurted out, "Hi there, can I speak to your lovely wife?"

"Sure, Loretta. She's right here." I smiled and handed the phone to Joyce. When Loretta called and got me, she typically visited for a few minutes before asking for her "lovely" daughter. So I figured the hurried request meant she had some important news to share. While Joyce and her mom talked, I started doing the dishes while listening to Joyce's half of the conversation, mostly only consisting of "Really!" or "Ah, hmm. Ah, hmm."

I enjoy my mother-in-law. I also admire her. Life has never been easy for Loretta, but she lives life easily because she takes such pleasure in it.

As the oldest child in a farm family, Loretta found herself saddled with all the work and responsibilities that her father had hoped to place on an oldest son. Somehow her father never got over the fact that his oldest child was not going to grow up to be a man. As a result, Loretta shouldered a heavy load from the start of her life. Her father acquired more and more land, and her workload grew proportionately. He was a driven man who pushed everyone around him just as hard. By age fifty, he grew close to fulfilling his ambitions. He got all the land he wanted, and it killed him.

By this time, Loretta had met Cliff, the boy from the farm next door. Like so many women during World War II, she worked, waited, and worried as Cliff fought at Normandy, through the hedge rows of France, and finally at the Battle of the Bulge. When he came home, they married.

Loretta bore fourteen children and had three miscarriages. The family lived out in the Wisconsin countryside in a house with no indoor plumbing, grew and canned much of its own food, and raised hogs and chickens for meat. Entertainment consisted of trips to the woods for berry-picking, bean fights in the garden, fierce games of sheep-head and blackjack, and periodic trips to the northern Wisconsin forests with as many kids as would fit into their one car. Every Sunday the Heils filled a pew at Mass at Saint Mary's Church. Life was simple, busy, and full.

Now, many people I know shake their heads when I tell them that Joyce's mom had fourteen children. The expression on their faces usually says, "That's impossible. How could any woman do that?" What particularly annoys me are expressions of pity, as if Loretta was a hapless victim of some male plot. Loretta's anything but a victim. She is one of the most alive people I know.

When Don, the youngest child, headed off to elementary school, everyone thought that Loretta would breathe a sigh of relief. Instead she grieved her empty nest. I'm sure that never having money to spare caused its problems, but I've never heard Loretta complain. Instead what I always hear are small triumphs of one of the kids or grandkids. Or how much she won playing blackjack at the local casino.

One time when Joyce and I were staying with her folks, we observed Loretta and Cliff playing a fierce game of blackjack. When she lost, Loretta would moan in despair as she passed her lost pennies over to Cliff. When she won, she fanned her breast and proclaimed, "I won! I won!" Cliff passed those same pennies back. She scooped them up as if she had won the state lottery.

Now that Joyce has lost a lot of weight, she has begun giving her mom clothes she can no longer wear. As soon as Joyce carries in the bags of garments, Mom hustles into the bedroom to try on her new wardrobe. I'll never forget Loretta sashaying around her living room in a red, wool, winter coat that Joyce gave her.

When the farmhouse in which they had raised their kids and had lived for scores of years began to crumble, Loretta and Cliff had to decide what to do. A new roof, new plumbing, and so on were out of the question. But this had been home. We wondered if Mom could leave her raspberry bushes, lush flower garden, rows of vegetables that had flourished under her care, and most of all the house full of memories.

Sure enough there were tears, but Loretta really took to life at the senior apartment. Now she drives her women friends to the beauty salon, plays cards with the crowd, and enjoys lunch at the senior center. As usual with Mom, life is good.

I heard Joyce hang up the phone just as I put the last dish in the drain. She was laughing. "What?" I asked. "Sounds like Mom won the lottery."

"Oh, it's better than the lottery. She won a jacket for Dad at the casino. It's celebrating some anniversary, so they're giving away door prizes. Mom won the jacket. You would swear it was a trip to Europe or the powerball drawing. My mom's something."

She is indeed, I thought, hoping that some day I would attain such wisdom, the wisdom that takes joy in simple gifts and offers gratitude for life's many pleasures.

Carl Koch

WHAT COUNTS ON YOUR PATH TO FULFILLMENT IS THAT WE REMEMBER THE GREAT TRUTH THAT MOMENTS OF SURPRISE WANT TO TEACH US: EVERYTHING IS GRATUITOUS, EVERY-THING IS GIFT. THE DEGREE TO WHICH WE ARE AWAKE TO THIS TRUTH IS THE MEASURE OF OUR GRATEFULNESS. AND GRATEFULNESS IS THE MEASURE OF OUR ALIVENESS.

David Steindl-Rast

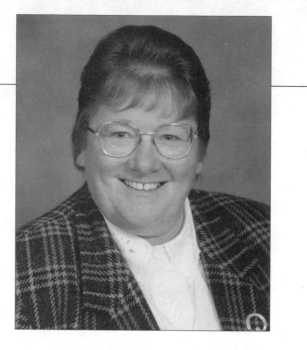

ANNE BRYAN SMOLLIN, C.S.J., lectures widely on wellness and spirituality. Both an educator and a therapist, she holds a Ph.D. in counseling from Walden University in Florida and is the executive director of the Counseling for Laity Center in Albany, New York.